EVELYN PARKER

....

The Frugal Renal Diet Cookbook for Beginners

How to Manage Chronic Kidney Disease (CKD) to Escape Dialysis. 21-Day Nutritional Plan for Progressive Renal Function Recovery. 301 Kidney-Friendly Recipes.

Chapter 6: Kidney-Friendly Fish & Seafood Recipes 140

Chapter 7: Kidney-Friendly Vegetables Recipes 172

Conclusion Errore. Il segnalibro non è definito.

The 21-Day Kidney Friendly Meal Plan

This meal plan is designed to provide you with the best healthy food for your kidneys. All these recipes are with clear instructions ahead. Try to eat one serving of these foods, but remember not to starve yourself. Enjoy.

Week 1

Monday (Day 1)

Breakfast: One Blueberry Muffin with Coffee or Tea

Lunch: Green Pesto Pasta

Snack: Half A Cup of Leached Broccoli

Dinner: Turmeric Lime Chicken

Tuesday (Day 2)

Breakfast: Two Maple Pancakes

Lunch: Quinoa Burger

Snack: A Few Slices of Apples

Dinner: Garlic Roasted Salmon & Brussels Sprouts

Wednesday (Day 3)

Breakfast: Blood Orange, Carrot, and Ginger Smoothie

Lunch: Cleansing Detox Soup

Snack: Half A Cup of Fresh Berries

Dinner: Turkey & Noodles

Thursday (Day 4)

Breakfast: One or two egg muffins

Lunch: Slow Cooker Cabbage Soup

Snack: 2,3 baby carrots with tea or coffee

Dinner: One Pot Greek Chicken and Lemon Rice

Friday (Day 5)

Breakfast: Loaded Veggie Eggs

Lunch: Chicken and Rice Soup

Snack: Few slices of pineapples

Dinner: Green Falafels

Saturday (Day 6)

Breakfast: Dilly Scrambled Eggs

Lunch: Vegan Meatloaf

Dinner: Turkey New Orleans style

Sunday (Day 7)

Breakfast: Homemade Buttermilk Pancake

Lunch: Pasta Soup

Snack: One Blueberry Muffin

Dinner: Roast Chicken with Turmeric and Fennel

Week 2

Monday (Day 8)

Breakfast: Easy Turkey Breakfast Burritos

Lunch: Capers pasta salad

Dinner: One-Pot Chicken and Dumplings

Tuesday (Day 9)

Breakfast: Diet Breakfast

Lunch: Cauliflower Soup

Dinner: Juicy Turkey Burgers with Zucchini

Wednesday (Day 10)

Breakfast: Egg Muffins

Lunch: Butternut Squash and Apple Soup

Snack: Half A Cup of Cherries

Dinner: Baked Pork Chops

Thursday (Day 11)

Breakfast: Quick and Easy Apple Oatmeal Custard

Lunch: Tofu Parmigiana

Snack: Low-Sodium Crackers

Dinner: Easy one-pot pasta

Friday (Day 12)

Breakfast: Microwave Coffee Cup Egg Scramble

Lunch: Pasta with Cauliflower

Snack: A Few Breadsticks

Dinner: Turmeric Lime Chicken

Saturday (Day 13)

Breakfast: Southwest Baked Egg Breakfast Cups

Lunch: Yucatan Lime Soup

Dinner: Turkey Chili

Sunday (Day 14)

Breakfast: Stuffed Breakfast Biscuits

Lunch: Healthy Pizza Pasta Salad

Snack: One Bagel with Coffee or Tea

Dinner: Spaghetti Squash Parmigiano

Week 3

Monday (Day 15)

Breakfast: Two Maple Pancakes

Lunch: Garlic Shells

Snack: Low Sodium Crackers

Dinner: Beef Stew

Tuesday (Day 16)

Breakfast: Mushroom & Red Pepper Omelet

Lunch: Broccoli Balls

Snack: Unsalted Pretzels

Dinner: Swordfish with Olives, Capers Polenta

Wednesday (Day 17)

Breakfast: Beach Boy Omelet

Lunch: Cauliflower Steaks

Snack: Few slices of apples

Dinner: Green Chili Stew

Thursday (Day 18)

Breakfast: Apple onion omelet

Lunch: Garbanzo Stir Fry

Snack: Animal crackers

Dinner: Seasoned Pork Chops

Friday (Day 19)

Breakfast: Quick and Easy Apple Oatmeal Custard

Lunch: Vegan Minestrone Soup

Dinner: Turmeric Lime Chicken

Saturday (Day 20)

Breakfast: No-Fuss Microwave Egg White French Toast

Lunch: Salmon with Lemon Caper Sauce

Snack: One blueberry muffin

Dinner: Pork Fajitas

Sunday (Day 21)

Breakfast: Apple Muffins

Lunch: Honey Garlic Chicken

Snack: One Bagel

Dinner: Vegan Minestrone Soup

Chapter 1: Kidney-Friendly Breakfast Recipes

1. Fluffy Homemade Buttermilk Pancake

Ingredients

- Olive oil: ¼ cup
- Low-fat buttermilk: 2 cups
- All-purpose flour: 2 cups
- Lemon juice: 1 teaspoon
- Sugar: 2 tablespoons
- 2 large eggs white
- Baking powder: one and a half teaspoons

Instructions

- Put a pan over medium flame.
- In a large bowl, add all the dry ingredients. In another bowl,

add oil, buttermilk, and egg whites mix and mix with dry ingredients.

- Mix it well.
- Spray oil on the pan. Pour the batter into the pan in a pancake shape.
- Cook until brown on both sides.
- Repeat with the rest of the batter, enjoy.

Nutrition Per Serving: Calories 217| Total Fat 9 g| Saturated Fat 1 g| Cholesterol 44 mg| Sodium 330 mg| Carbohydrates 27 g|Protein 6 g|Phosphorus 100 mg|Potassium 182 mg| Fiber 1 g| Calcium 74 mg

1.2 Blueberry Muffins

Ingredients

- 2 and a half cups fresh blueberries
- Half cup low-fat unsalted butter
- One and 1/4 cups of artificial sweetener
- Soy milk: 2 cups
- All-purpose flour: 2 cups
- Half teaspoon of salt
- Three eggs' white
- Baking powder: 2 teaspoons

Instructions

- In a food mixer, add sugar alternative and margarine, blend it on low until smooth.

- Add eggs, mix until combined well.

- Add dry ingredients after sifting, and add milk.

- Take half a cup of berries and mash them. Mix in the mixture with your clean hands. Add the rest of the berries.

- Spray oil on the muffin cups.

- Pour muffin mixture into muffin cups.

- Bake in the oven for half an hour at 375° F.

Nutrition Per Serving: Calories 275| Total Fat 9 g| Saturated Fat 5 g| Cholesterol 53 mg| Sodium 210 mg| Carbohydrates 44 g| Protein 5 g| Phosphorus 100 mg| Potassium 121 mg| Dietary Fiber 1.3 g| Calcium 108 mg

1.3 Easy Turkey Breakfast Burritos

Ingredients

- ¼ cup of chopped bell peppers

- 4 cups of ground turkey

- ¼ cup of olive oil

- 8 egg whites, whisked

- ¼ cup of chopped onions

- Half teaspoon of chili powder

- Jalapeño peppers(seeded): 2 tablespoons

- Eight pieces of flour burrito shells

- Scallions: 2 tablespoons, diced

- Half teaspoon of smoked paprika

- 1 cup shredded vegan cheese

Instructions

- In a pan over medium heat, sauté peppers, cilantro, turkey, scallions, and onions. Until translucent.

- In another pan, cook the whisked eggs.

- In burrito, add turkey and vegetable mix, eggs, and cheese.

- Fold and serve.

Nutrition Per Serving: Calories 407| Total Fat 24 g| Saturated Fat 7 g| Trans Fat 0 g| Cholesterol 237 mg| Sodium 513 mg| Carbohydrates 23 g| Protein 25 g| Phosphorus 359 mg |Potassium 285 mg| Dietary Fiber 2 g| Calcium 209 mg

1.4 Loaded Veggie Eggs

Ingredients

- 1/4 cup of diced onion

- 6-7 whites of eggs

- 3 cups of fresh kale

- One clove of pressed garlic

- Oil: 1 tbsp.

- 1/4 cup of diced bell pepper

- One cup of cauliflower

- Black pepper: 1/4 tsp

- Spring onion for garnish

Instructions

- Whisk the egg whites.

- In a pan, over medium flame, add peppers and onions in the pan and sauté for three minutes.

- Then add garlic and cauliflower—Cook well on low heat for five minutes.

- Add egg whites, mix with vegetables.

- When eggs are cooked, garnish with spring onion, black pepper.

- Serve hot.

Nutrition Per Serving: Calories 240| Total Fat 16.6g| Cholesterol 372mg| Sodium 195mg| Total Carbohydrate 7.8g| Dietary Fiber 2.7g| Protein 15.3g| Potassium 605.2mg| Phosphorus 253.6mg

1.5 Diet Breakfast

Ingredients

- 3 egg whites
- Garlic: 1/4 tsp, minced
- Bell pepper: 2 tbsp. Chopped
- Cabbage: 1/4 cup, chopped
- Mushrooms: 1/4 cup
- Black pepper
- Jalapeno: 2 tbsp. chopped

Instructions

- In a saucepan, sauté all ingredients, add the mushroom in the last.

- Do not overcook vegetables.

- Then add pepper and garlic to eggs.

- Scramble on Low Heat.

- Sprinkle with basil and serve

Nutrients per serving: Calories 176 | Protein 7.3 g |Carbohydrates 9.2 g |Fat 8.2 g |Cholesterol 132 mg |Sodium 162 mg |Potassium 211 mg| Phosphorus 115 mg |Calcium 17.4 mg |Fiber 3 g

1.6 Breakfast Burrito

Ingredients

- 2 flour tortillas
- 4 egg whites
- Green chilies: 3 tablespoons chopped
- Half tsp. Of hot pepper sauce
- Ground cumin: 1/4 teaspoon

Instructions

- In a skillet over medium flame, spray cooking oil.

- In a mixing bowl, add eggs, cumin, green chilies, hot sauce, and whisk well.

- Add whisked eggs into skillet. Let it cook for two minutes until eggs are cooked.

- Now, lay burritos on a hot skillet and or microwave them and place egg mixture on them.

- Roll and fold on sides.

- Serve hot

Nutrients per serving: Calories 366|Protein 18 g| Carbohydrates 33 g| Fat 18 g| Cholesterol 372 mg| Sodium

394 mg| potassium 215 mg| Phosphorus 254 mg| Calcium 117 mg| Fiber 2.5 g

1.7 Maple Pancakes

Ingredients

- 1% low-fat milk: 1 cup
- All-purpose flour: 1 cup
- Honey: 1 tablespoon
- Salt: two pinches
- Maple extract: 1 tablespoon
- Egg whites: 2 large
- Baking powder: 2 teaspoons
- Olive oil: 2 tablespoons

Instructions

- In a mixing bowl, mix flour, baking powder, salt. Mix well.
- Set it aside.
- In a big mixing bowl, mix egg whites, oil, maple extract, honey, and milk.
- Now mix dry ingredients and wet ingredients. Do not over mix. It should be lumpy.
- Put a skillet over medium flame, spray cooking oil and pour the batter and cook pancakes until brown on both sides.
- Serve hot

Nutrients per serving: Calories 178|Protein 6 g| Carbohydrates 25 g| Fat 6 g| Cholesterol 2 mg| Sodium 267 mg| Potassium 126 mg| Phosphorus 116 mg| Calcium 174 mg| Fiber 0.7 g|

1.8 Mini Frittatas

Ingredients

- Low fat shredded cheese: ¼ cup
- Red bell pepper: ⅓ cup chopped
- Zucchini: ⅓ cup chopped
- Broccoli: ⅓ cup diced
- Fresh basil: 2-3 tbsp.
- Pepper: ¼ tsp
- Seasoning(salt-free): half tbsp.
- 10-12 eggs' whites and 3 yolks

Instructions

- Let the oven Preheat to 375 degrees.
- Spray the muffin pan with oil.
- In a mixing bowl, mix zucchini, basil, red bell pepper, and broccoli.
- In another bowl, mix pepper, cheese, seasoning (salt-free), eggs, and salt.
- Mix the egg mix to vegetables.
- Pour the egg mixture into muffin cups, at least 1/3 cup.
- Bake for 18-20 minutes at 375 F or until cooked.
- Serve right away.

Nutrients per serving: Calories 245 | Protein 11 g |Carbohydrates 9.2 g |Fat 7.7 g |Cholesterol 121 mg |Sodium 99.2 mg |Potassium 201 mg| Phosphorus 109 mg |Calcium 27.9 mg |Fiber 2 g

1.9 Dilly Scrambled Eggs

Ingredients

- Dried dill weed: 1 teaspoon
- Three large egg white
- Crumbled goat cheese: 1 table-spoon
- Black pepper: 1/8 teaspoon

Instructions

- In a bowl, mix eggs.
- Pour the egg mixture into the skillet over medium flame.
- Sprinkle dill weed and black pepper to eggs.
- Cook until eggs are done.
- Garnish with goat cheese.
- Serve right away.

Nutrients per serving: Calories 194|Protein 16 g| Carbohydrates 1 g| Fat 14 g| Cholesterol 334 mg| Sodium 213 mg| Potassium 162 mg| Phosphorus 50 mg| Calcium 214 mg| Fiber 0.2 g

1.10 Start Your Day Bagel

Ingredients

- 1 bagel
- Two red onion slices
- Low fat cream cheese: 2 table-spoons
- Lemon-pepper seasoning(low-sodium): 1 teaspoon
- Two small tomato slices

Instructions

- Slice the bagel and toast to your liking
- Spread cream cheese on each half bagel.
- Add tomato slice, onion slice.
- Sprinkle with lemon pepper.

Nutrients per serving: Calories 134|Protein 5 g| Carbohydrates 19 g| Fat 6 g| Cholesterol 15 mg| Sodium 219 mg| Potassium 162 mg| Phosphorus 50 mg| calcium 9 mg| Fiber 1.6 g

1.11 Egg Muffins

Ingredients

- Ten large eggs whites
- bell peppers: 1 cup
- 2 cups ground pork
- Onion: 1 cup
- Garlic minced: half teaspoon
- Half teaspoon of herb seasoning
- Poultry seasoning (no salt): 1/4 teaspoon
- Salt: two pinches or to taste
- Milk substitute: 2 tablespoons

Instructions

- Let the oven preheat to 350° F and spray cooking oil on the muffin tin
- Chop the vegetables finely.
- In a bowl, mix garlic pork, herb seasoning, poultry seasoning to make sausage.

- In a skillet, cook the sausage until done and drain the liquid if any
- Whisk the eggs with salt and milk.
- Add vegetables and sausage crumbles, mix well.
- Add egg mixture into muffin tins, leave some space on top.
- Bake for 18 to 20 minutes or until done.
- Serve hot.

Nutrients per serving: Calories 154|Protein 12 g| Carbohydrates 3 g| Fat 10 g| Cholesterol 230 mg| Sodium 155 mg| Potassium 200 mg| Phosphorus 154 mg| Calcium 37 mg| Fiber 0.5 g

1.12 Quick & Easy Apple Oatmeal Custard

Ingredients

- Half cup of almond milk
- Quick-cooking oatmeal: 1/3 cup
- Cinnamon: 1/4 teaspoon
- Half apple
- Two egg white

Instructions

- Finely diced the half apple.
- In a large mug, add almond milk, egg, and oats. Mix well with a fork.
- Add apple and cinnamon. Mix well.

- Microwave for two minutes, on high.
- Fluff it with a fork.
- Cook for another sixty-second if required.
- Add in little milk or water if the consistency is too thick.

Nutrients per serving: Calories 248|Protein 11 g| Carbohydrates 33 g| Fat 8 g| Cholesterol 186 mg| Sodium 164 mg| Potassium 362 mg| phosphorus 240 mg| Calcium 154 mg| Fiber 5.8 g

1.13 Microwave Coffee Cup Egg Scramble

Ingredients

- 1% low-fat milk: 2 tablespoons
- 1 large egg+ 2 whites

Instructions

- Spray the coffee cup with oil. Add eggs and milk and whisk.
- Put the coffee cup in the microwave, let it cook for 45 seconds, then remove and fluff with a fork.
- Cook for an additional 30-45 seconds, until eggs are almost done.
- Add pepper and enjoy.

Nutrients per serving: Calories 117|Protein 15 g| Carbohydrates 3 g| Fat 5 g| Cholesterol 188 mg| Sodium 194 mg| Potassium 226 mg| Phosphorus 138 mg| Calcium 72 mg| Fiber 0 g

1.14 No-Fuss Microwave Egg White French Toast

Ingredients

- Half cup of egg whites
- One slice of bread
- Sugar-free syrup: 2 tablespoons
- Unsalted butter: 1 teaspoon, softened

Instructions

- Add bread to slice. Cut into cubes.
- Add cubed slices into a bowl.
- Add egg whites over bread pieces
- Add syrup on top. Microwave for 60 seconds or more until eggs are set.

Nutrients per serving: Calories 200 |Protein 15 g|Carbohydrates 24 g|Fat 5 g|Cholesterol 11 mg|Sodium 415 mg|Potassium 235 mg|Phosphorus 54 mg|Calcium 50 mg|Fiber 0.7 g

1.15 Easy Turkey Breakfast Burritos

Ingredients

- 8 flour burritos
- 4 cups of ground turkey
- Olive oil: ¼ cup
- Diced onions: ¼ cup
- Bell peppers: ¼ cup chopped
- Fresh scallions: 2 tablespoons, chopped
- 9 whisked egg white
- Jalapeño peppers(seeded): 2 tablespoons
- Fresh cilantro
- Smoked paprika: half teaspoon
- Chili powder: half teaspoon
- Vegan shredded cheese: 1 cup

Instructions

- In a skillet, sauté scallions, turkey, cilantro, peppers, and onions. Add in spices and mix well. turn off the heat
- In another pan, on medium flame, add oil and eggs. Cook well
- In a burrito shell, add vegetables and meatloaf mix, add eggs and cheese in burrito shells.
- Fold on sides and serve.

Nutrition Per Serving: Calories 407 Cal| Total Fat 24 g|Saturated Fat 7 g| Trans Fat 0 g|Cholesterol 237 mg|Sodium 513 mg|Carbohydrates 23 g| Protein 25 g|Phosphorus 359 mg|Potassium 285 mg|Dietary Fiber 2 g| Calcium 209 mg

1.16 Tofu Scrambler

Ingredients

- Onion powder: 1 teaspoon
- Olive oil: 1 teaspoon
- Green bell pepper: ¼ cup diced
- Red bell pepper: ¼ cup diced
- Turmeric: ⅛ teaspoon

- Firm tofu: 1 cup (less than 10% calcium)
- 2 clove garlic, minced

Instructions

- In a non-stick pan, add bell peppers and garlic in olive oil.
- Rinse the tofu, and add in skillet break it into pieces with hands.
- Add all the remaining ingredients.
- Stir often, and cook on medium flame until the tofu becomes a light golden brown, for almost 20 minutes.
- Serve warm.

Nutrition Per Serving: Calories 213 Cal| Total Fat 13 g| Saturated Fat 2 g| Trans Fat 0 g|Cholesterol 0 mg|Sodium 24 mg|Carbohydrates 10 g |Protein 18 g|Phosphorus 242 mg|Potassium 467 mg|Dietary Fiber 2 g|Calcium 274 mg

1.17 Southwest Baked Egg Breakfast Cups

Ingredients

- Rice: 3 cups, cooked
- Half cup of shredded cheddar cheese
- Half cup of chopped green chilies
- 1/4 cups of cherry peppers diced
- Half cup of skim milk
- 3 egg whites whisked
- Ground cumin: half teaspoon
- Black pepper: half teaspoon

Instructions

- In a bowl, mix chilies, cherry peppers, eggs, cumin, 2 ounces of cheese, rice, black pepper.
- Spray the muffin tins with oil
- Pour mix into muffins tin. Garnish with cheese.
- Bake for 15 minutes at 400° F or until set.

Nutrition Per Serving: Calories 109 cal|Total Fat 4 g|Saturated Fat 2 g| Trans Fat 0 g|Cholesterol 41 mg|Sodium 79 mg|Carbohydrates 13 g|Protein 5 g|Phosphorus 91 mg|Potassium 82 mg|Dietary Fiber 0.5 g|Calcium 91 mg

1.18 Stuffed Breakfast Biscuits

Ingredients

- Baking powder: half teaspoon
- Honey: 1 tablespoon
- Lemon juice: 1 tablespoon
- Softened unsalted butter: 8 tablespoons
- Milk: ¾ cup
- Flour: 2 cups

Filling

- Cheddar cheese: 1 cup shredded
- Five egg white
- Scallions: ¼ cup, thinly sliced
- 1 cup chopped bacon (reduced-sodium)

Instructions

- Let the oven Preheat to 425° F.

For Filling

- Cook the eggs, scrambled
- Cook bacon to crisp.
- Mix filling ingredients and set it aside

The Dough

- In a big bowl, add all the dry ingredients.
- Add in butter and cut with a fork, and add in lemon juice and milk. Knead well.
- Spray muffin tin with oil generously.
- Pour ¼ cup of mixture into the muffin tins.
- Bake for 10-12 minutes at 425° F until golden brown.

Nutrition Per Serving: Calories 330 cal|Total Fat 23 g|Saturated Fat 11 g|Trans Fat 0.6 g|Cholesterol 105 mg|Sodium 329 mg|Carbohydrates 19 g|Protein 11 g|Phosphorus 170 mg|Potassium 152 mg|Dietary Fiber 1 g|Calcium 107 mg

1.19 Cheesesteak Quiche

Ingredients

- Olive oil: 2 tablespoons
- 2 cups of trimmed sirloin steak, roughly chopped
- Onions: 1 cup, chopped
- Cheese: Half cup, shredded
- Six egg white whisked
- Ground black pepper: half teaspoon
- Low-fat Cream: 1 cup
- Par-cooked prepared piecrust

Instructions

- In a pan with oil, Sauté onions, and chopped steak. Cook until meat is cooked. Let it cool for ten minutes. Mix in cheese set it aside.
- In a bowl, whisk cream eggs with black pepper, mix it well.
- Add cheese mix and steak on pie crust, then add the egg mixture on top and half an hour bake at 350° F.
- and turn off the oven and Cover the quiche with foil.
- Let it sit for ten minutes, then serve.

Nutrition Per Serving: Calories 527 cal|Total Fat 19 g|Saturated Fat 17 g|Trans Fat 1 g|Cholesterol 240 mg|Sodium 392 mg|Carbohydrates 22 g|Protein 22 g|Phosphorus 281 mg|Potassium 308 mg|Dietary Fiber 1 g|Calcium 137 mg

1.20 Chocolate Pancakes with Moon Pie Stuffing

Ingredients

Moon Pie Stuffing

- Heavy cream: ¼ cup

- Cocoa powder(unsweetened): 1 tablespoon
- Half cup of low fat softened cream cheese
- Honey: 2 tbsp.

Chocolate Pancakes

- One large egg white
- Flour: 1 cup
- Cocoa powder(unsweetened): 3 tablespoons
- Half teaspoon baking powder
- Olive oil: 2 tablespoons
- Lemon juice: 1 tablespoon
- Honey: 3 tablespoons
- Vanilla extract: 2 teaspoons
- Almond milk: 1 cup

Instructions

Moon Pie Filling

- Beat cocoa and heavy cream together until stiff peaks are formed.
- Whip in cream cheese, marshmallow cream, and whey protein powder for about a minute or until well blended, but don't overbeat. Cover and set aside in the fridge.

Pancakes

- Mix all the dry ingredients in a large bowl and set aside.
- Mix all the wet ingredients in a medium-size bowl.

- Slowly fold in wet ingredients to the dry ingredients just until wet, but don't over mix.
- Cook the pancakes on a lightly oiled griddle on medium heat or 375° F.
- Use about 1/8 cup of batter to form 4-inch pancakes, flipping when they start to bubble.

Nutrition Per Serving: Calories 194 Cal |Total Fat 9 g|Saturated Fat 4 g|Trans Fat 0 g|Cholesterol 36 mg|Sodium 121 mg| Carbohydrates 22 g| Protein 7 g| Phosphorus 134 mg|Potassium 135 mg|Dietary Fiber 1 g|Calcium 67 mg

1.21 Apple Muffins

Ingredients

- One and a half tsp of cinnamon
- One and a half cup of raw apple
- Half cup of water
- 1 cup honey
- Half cup olive oil
- 2 large egg white
- Vanilla: 1 tbsp.
- One and a half cup all-purpose white flour
- Baking powder: 1 tsp

Instructions

- Let the oven preheat to 400 F. add muffin papers in a muffin tin.
- Peel and chop the apple into small pieces.

- In a bowl, whisk eggs with water, honey, oil, vanilla and mix well
- In another bowl, mix baking powder, one teaspoon cinnamon, flour.
- Sift the flour mixture into the egg mix.
- The batter should be lumpy. Add in the apple pieces.
- Pour batter into muffin cups, sprinkle cinnamon on top.
- Enjoy warm.

Nutrition per serving: Sodium 177 mg|Protein 3 g|Potassium 46 mg|Phosphorus 34 mg |Calcium 10 mg|Calories 162 kcal|Fat 10 g| Water 60 g |Carbohydrates 15 g

1.22 Breakfast Casserole

Ingredients

- 1% low-fat milk: 1 cup
- One cup of pork sausage (reduced-fat)
- Five large egg whites
- Half teaspoon dry mustard
- One cup of cream cheese (low fat)
- Half chopped onion
- White bread, cut into cubes: 4 slices

Instructions

- Let the oven preheat to 325 F
- Break the sausage and cook in a pan, set it aside

- In a blender, pulse the rest of the ingredients. Do not add bread yet.
- Add the cooked sausage to the mix.
- In a 9 by 9 dish, add the bread, and add sausage mix on top
- Bake for 55 minutes.
- Serve hot and enjoy.

Nutrients per serving: Calories 224 | Protein 11 g| Carbohydrates 9 g| Fat 16 g| Cholesterol 149 mg| Sodium 356 mg|Potassium 201 mg| Phosphorus 159 mg|Calcium 97 mg |fiber 0.4 g|

1.23 Apple Onion Omelet

Ingredients

- Butter: 1 tablespoon
- Three large egg whites
- Water: 1 tablespoon
- Black pepper: 1/8 teaspoon
- 1% low-fat milk: 1/4 cup
- Shredded cheddar cheese: 2 tablespoons
- Sweet onion: 3/4 cup
- One big apple

Instructions

- Let the oven Preheat to 400° F.
- Peel and clean apple. Thinly slice the onion and apples
- In a bowl, whisk the egg with milk, pepper, water. Set it aside.

- In a pan, over a low flame, melt the butter.
- Add apple and onion to the butter, cook for five minutes.
- Add egg mix on top cook on medium flame until the edges are set.
- Add the cheese on the top.
- Put the skillet in the oven and bake for 10-12 minutes, or until set.
- Serve hot

Nutrients per serving: calories 284 | Protein 13 | Carbohydrates 22 | Fat 16 | Cholesterol 303| Sodium 169| potassium 341|Phosphorus 238 |Calcium 147 |Fiber 3.5

1.24 Beach Boy Omelet

Ingredients

- Green bell pepper: 2 tablespoons, chopped
- Canola oil: 1 teaspoon
- Hash browns: 2 tablespoons (shredded)
- Soy milk: 2 tablespoons
- One egg and two egg whites
- Onion: 2 tablespoons, chopped

Instructions

- In a pan, heat oil over medium flame. Sauté green pepper and onion for two minutes
- Then add hash browns, cook for five minutes.

- Whisk eggs with non-dairy creamer or soy milk
- In another pan, cook the eggs until set.
- Add the hash brown mixture in the center of eggs, wrap with eggs and serve

Nutrients per serving: Calories 228 | Protein 15 g |Carbohydrates 12 g |Fat 13 g |Cholesterol 165 mg |Sodium 180 mg |Potassium 307 mg|Phosphorus 128 mg |Calcium 38 mg |Fiber 0.9 g

1.25 Mushroom & Red Pepper Omelet

Ingredients

- Half cup raw mushroom
- 3 large egg white
- Onion: 2 tablespoons
- Red peppers: 1/4 cup
- Whipped cream cheese: 2 tablespoons
- Butter: 2 teaspoons
- Black pepper: 1/4 teaspoon

Instructions

- Chop up the red peppers, onion, and mushroom
- In a pan, melt the butter (one tsp.). Sauté red peppers, onion, and mushroom. Set it aside.
- Melt another tsp. of butter in a pan. Cook eggs. When eggs are half cooked, pour vegetable mix with cream cheese on top. Cook eggs until set

- Continue cooking until eggs are set.
- Fold the half omelet on top of the cream cheese mix. Add black pepper and serve

Nutrients per serving: Calories 178 | Protein 8.8 g |Carbohydrates 8.2 g |Fat 6.7 g |Cholesterol 132 mg |Sodium 156 mg |Potassium 201 mg|Phosphorus 121 mg |Calcium 21 mg |Fiber 0.4 g

Chapter 2: Kidney-Friendly Soup Recipes

2.1 Spring Vegetable Soup

Ingredients

- Vegetable broth(low-sodium): 4 cups
- Fresh green beans: 1 cup
- Half cup carrots
- Celery: 3/4 cup
- Garlic powder: 1 teaspoon
- Half cup onion
- Half cup mushrooms
- Olive oil: 2 tablespoons
- Dried oregano leaves: 1 teaspoon
- 1/4 teaspoon salt
- Half cup frozen corn

Instructions

- Trim the green beans and chop into two-inch pieces
- Chop up the vegetables.

- In a pot, heat olive oil, sauté the onion and celery, till tender.
- Then add the remaining ingredients.
- Let it boil. Lower the heat, let it simmer.
- Cook for almost an hour.

Nutrients per serving: Calories 114| Protein 2 g| Carbohydrates 13 g| Fat 6 g| Cholesterol 0 mg| Sodium 262 mg| Potassium 365 mg| Phosphorus 108 mg| Calcium 48 mg| Fiber 3.4 g|

2.2 Kidney Diet Friendly Chicken Noodle Soup

Ingredients

- One cup cooked Chicken Breast
- Unsalted Butter: 1 tbsp.
- Half cup of Chopped Celery
- Chicken Stock: 5 cups
- Half tsp Ground Basil
- Half cup of chopped Onions
- Ground Black Pepper: 1/4 tsp
- Egg Noodles: 2 cups, Dry
- Sliced Carrots: 1 cup
- Half tsp Ground Oregano

Instructions

- Chop up all the vegetables.
- In a Dutch oven (5 quarts), melt butter over low heat—Cook celery and onion for five minutes. Add in the carrots, oregano, chicken stock, basil, pepper, chicken and, noodles.

- Let it boil. Lower the heat and let it simmer for 20 minutes.
- Serve hot.

Nutrition per serving: Calories: 186| Protein: 15.8 g| Carbohydrate: 19.7 g| Dietary Fiber: 1.461 g| Phosphorus: 178.8 mg| Potassium: 478.9 mg| Sodium: 327.2 mg|

2.3 Renal-Friendly Cream of Mushroom Soup

Ingredients

- Minced mushrooms: 1/4 cup
- Unsalted butter: 3 tbsp.
- All-purpose flour: 2 and a half tbsp.
- Sea salt, pepper to taste
- Low sodium chicken broth: half cup
- Finely chopped onion: 1/4 cup
- Unsweetened almond milk: half cup

Instructions

- In a skillet, melt the butter and sauté onions till tender
- Add mushrooms and cook for five minutes. Add flour and cook for one minute or a few seconds more
- Add in milk and broth mix continuously.
- Let it simmer until it becomes thick for five minutes.

Nutrition per serving: Total Fat 18.2g| Cholesterol 45.8mg| Sodium 162.8mg| Total Carbohydrate 10.2g| Dietary Fiber 0.9g| Protein 2.1g| Iron 1mg| Potassium 123.7mg

2.4 Rotisserie Chicken Noodle Soup

Ingredients

- Carrots: 1 cup, sliced
- One cooked rotisserie chicken
- Half cup of onion, chopped
- Celery: 1 cup, sliced
- Chicken broth(low-sodium): 8 cups
- Fresh parsley: 3 tablespoons
- Wide noodles: 6 ounces, uncooked

Instructions

- Take the bones out of the chicken and cut into one-inch pieces. Take four cups of chicken pieces.
- In a large pot, add chicken broth let it boil.
- Add noodles, chicken, and vegetables to the broth.
- Let it boil, and cook for 15 minutes. Make sure noodles are tender.
- Serve with chopped parsley on top.

Nutrients per serving: Calories 185| Protein 21 g| Carbohydrates 14 g| Fat 5 g| Cholesterol 63 mg| Sodium 361 mg|

Potassium 294 mg| Phosphorus 161 mg | Calcium 22 mg| Fiber 1.4 g

2.5 Quick & Easy Ground Beef Soup

Ingredients

- Frozen mixed vegetables: 3 cups
- Half cup of onion, chopped
- Beef broth(reduced-sodium): 1 cup
- White rice: 1/3 cup, uncooked
- Lemon pepper (no salt): 2 teaspoons, seasoning
- 4 cups of lean ground beef
- Sour cream: 1 tablespoon
- Water: 2 cups

Instructions

- In a pot, sauté onion, brown the beef. Drain the fat.
- Add all the remaining ingredients and seasoning.
- Let it boil. Lower the heat, cover it, and cook for half an hour.
- Turn off the heat, add sour cream.

Nutrients per serving: calories 222 | Protein 20 g| Carbohydrates 19 g| Fat 8 g| Cholesterol 52 mg| Sodium 170 mg| Potassium 448 mg| Phosphorus 210 mg| Calcium 43 mg| Fiber 4.3 g

2.6 Chicken & Dill Soup

Ingredients

- One chicken whole
- Carrots, 1 pound, sliced
- Low-sodium veggie stock for 6 cups
- One cup of yellow, diced onion
- A pinch of black pepper and Salt
- Two dill teaspoons, diced
- Half cup red, minced onion

Instructions

- Place the chicken in a saucepan, add the water to coat it. Let it simmer for 1 hour.
- Take chicken out, remove the bones, strip the meat, strain the soup, put everything back in the saucepan, hot it over a moderate flame, and add the chicken.
- Add the carrots, red onion, a pinch of Salt, yellow onion, black pepper, and dill, roast for fifteen minutes, and put in bowls.

Nutrients per serving: Calories 295| Protein 21 g| Carbohydrates 28 g| Fat 11 g| Cholesterol 45 mg| Sodium 385 mg| Potassium 312 mg| Phosphorus 252 mg| Calcium 183 mg | Fiber 3.3 g

2.7 Maryland's Eastern Shore Cream of Crab Soup

Ingredients

- 1 cup non-dairy creamer
- Unsalted butter: 1 tablespoon
- Old bay seasoning: 1/4 teaspoon
- 2 cups crab meat

- Chicken broth(low-sodium): 4 cups
- One medium onion
- Cornstarch: 2 tablespoons
- Black pepper: 1/8 teaspoon
- Dill weed: 1/8 teaspoon

Instructions

- In a large pot, melt butter over medium flame.
- Add chopped onion to the pot. Cook until tender.
- Add crab meat—Cook for 2 to 3 minutes. Stir often.
- Add chicken broth, let it boil. Turn heat down to low.
- Mix starch and creamer in a bowl. Mix well.
- Add the mixture to the soup, increase the heat, stir until the soup thickens and gets to a boil.
- Add Old Bay, dill weed, pepper to soup.

Nutrients per serving: Calories 130 | Protein 12 g| carbohydrates 7 g| Fat 6 g| Cholesterol 53 mg| sodium 212 mg| Potassium 312 mg| Phosphorus 80 mg| Calcium 86 mg|Fiber 0.4 g

2.8 Old Fashioned Salmon Soup

Ingredients

- Chicken broth, reduced-sodium: 2 cups
- Unsalted butter: 2 tablespoons
- Half cup of onion, chopped
- Sockeye salmon: 1 pound, cooked
- One medium carrot, chopped
- 1% low-fat milk: 2 cups
- Half cup of celery, chopped
- Black pepper: 1/8 teaspoon
- Water: 1/4 cup
- Cornstarch: 1/4 cup

Instructions

- In a large pot, melt the butter and cook the vegetables on low, medium flame until tender.
- Add the cooked salmon chunks. Add in the milk, broth, pepper.
- Let it simmer on low heat.
- Mix water and cornstarch. Keep stirring and slowly add the corn starch mix. Cook until soup becomes thick.
- Simmer for 5 minutes and serve.

Nutrients per serving: Calories 155| Protein 14 g| Carbohydrates 9 g| Fat 7 g| Cholesterol 37 mg| Sodium 113 mg| Potassium 369 mg| Phosphorus 218 mg| Calcium 92 mg| Fiber 0.5 g

2.9 Turkey, Wild Rice, & Mushroom Soup

Ingredients

- Turkey: 2 cups, cooked, shredded
- Half cup of onion, chopped
- Half cup of carrots, chopped

- Two garlic cloves, minced
- Chicken broth, low-sodium: 5 cups
- Half cup of red bell pepper, chopped
- Half cup of uncooked wild rice,
- Olive oil: 1 tablespoon
- Half teaspoon salt
- Two bay leaves
- Herb seasoning: 1/4 teaspoon
- Dried thyme: 1-and half teaspoon
- Black pepper: 1/4 teaspoon
- Half cup of sliced mushrooms

Instructions

- In a pot, boil the one and ¾ broth over medium flame. Add rice to the broth and cook. Let it boil. Turn the heat down. Cover it and let it simmer until all broth is absorbed.
- In a Dutch oven, heat oil, add garlic, bell pepper, onion, and carrots. Sauté them.
- Add the mushroom to the vegetables, then add the broth, turkey, herb seasoning, salt, pepper, thyme, and bay leaves. Cook until it is well heated. Stir often.
- Before adding the rice, take out the bay leaves. Cook for a minute and serve.

Nutrition per serving: Calories 210| Protein 23 g| Carbohydrates 15 g| Fat 5 g| Cholesterol 35 mg| Sodium 270 mg| Potassium 380 mg| Phosphorus 200 mg| Calcium 32 mg| Fiber 2.3 g

2.10 Slow Cooker Kale & Turkey Meatball Soup

Ingredients

- 4 cups of ground turkey
- Bread: 2 slices
- Kale: 4 cups
- ¼ of a cup milk
- 2 cloves of garlic pressed
- One medium shallot finely diced
- ½ of a teaspoon freshly grated nutmeg
- One teaspoon of oregano
- 1/4 of a teaspoon red pepper flakes
- Italian parsley chopped: 2 tablespoons
- 2 carrots cut into slices
- One egg white
- One tablespoon of olive oil
- Chicken or vegetable broth: 8 cups
- Half yellow onion finely diced
- Half of a cup Parmigiano-Reggiano grated, extra for garnish
- Kosher salt and freshly ground pepper

Instructions

- In a large mixing bowl, add milk, cut the bread into pieces, and let it soak in milk. Add the garlic, turkey, nutmeg, shallot, red pepper flakes, salt, oregano, pepper, egg, cheese, and parsley. Mix carefully with your hands. Use a scooper to make half-inch balls.

- Put a wide skillet on medium flame, heat the olive oil, then sear the meatballs gently on every side for two minutes. Turn off the heat and set it aside.

- Add the onion, stock, kale, and carrots to a 5 to 7 quarter slow cooker.

- Add meatballs the kale, and cook for four hours at low or until the meatballs start floating to the top.

- Garnish the soup with Parmesan grated cheese, red pepper flakes, and fresh leaves of parsley.

Nutrition per serving: 250 calories| total fat 23g |carbohydrates 20.3g | protein 14.4g| Cholesterol 25 mg| Sodium 214 mg| Potassium 276 mg| Phosphorus 198 mg| Calcium 28.8 mg| Fiber 2.8 g

2.11 Greek Lemon Chicken Soup

Ingredients

- Boneless: 4 cups of skinless chicken thighs, cut into bite-size pieces

- Chicken broth: 8 cups

- Kale: 4 cups

- Extra-virgin olive oil: 2 tablespoons, divided

- Freshly ground black pepper and Kosher salt

- Three carrots peeled, finely diced

- 2 stalks of celery finely chopped

- 4 cloves of pressed garlic

- Half teaspoon of dried thyme

- Two bay leaves

- Sliced fresh dill: 2 tablespoons

- One cup cubed sweet potatoes

- One onion finely chopped

- Squeezed lemon juice: 2 tablespoons(fresh)or more, if needed

- Sliced fresh parsley leaves: 2 tablespoons

Instruction

- Put a large saucepan or Dutch oven over medium flame and add one tablespoon of olive oil.

- Season the chicken thighs with black pepper and fine salt to your liking. Add the seasoned chicken things to the pan and cook for about three minutes; until golden brown, set it aside.

- Add the remaining one tablespoon of olive oil in the separate pan, with celery, garlic, onion, and carrots, stir frequently, and let it cook for about four minutes.

- Add in thyme, cook for about one minute, until fragrant.

- Then stir in the bay leaves and chicken stock, let it boil. Add in chicken and potatoes, stir and cook for 15 minutes, till soup is thickened.

- Add in the kale, cook for two minutes, till wilted. Add in parsley, dill, and lemon juice

- Season with salt and black pepper, to your taste.

- Serve hot, and enjoy

Nutrition per serving: Calories 243 g| Total Fat 9.0g|Carbohydrate 18.0g|Protein 19.0g |Cholesterol 18.2 mg| Sodium 198 mg| Potassium 213 mg| Phosphorus 187 mg| Calcium 29.2 mg| Fiber 2.5 g

2.12 Lemon Chicken Soup

Ingredients

- Eggs: 3 large whites

- Chicken broth: 6 cups

- Shredded and cooked chicken breast:1 cup

- Fresh lemon juice:1/4 cup

- Kosher Salt and freshly ground black pepper (to taste.)

- Orzo:1 cup

Instructions

- Add chicken stock to a big saucepan and let it boil.

- Add in orzo, cook until soft to your liking.

- Mix eggs and lemon juice.

- When orzo is cooked to your liking, take out one cup of chicken broth and add in egg mix one tablespoon at a time. Mixing constantly

- Then add this egg mixture back into the broth, constantly stirring.

- Add the cooked shredded chicken in the broth, let it simmer until the soup becomes thick, often stirring, for about five minutes.

- Add salt and freshly ground black pepper to taste.

Nutrition per serving: Calories 451|Carbs: 42g| Protein: 32g |Fat: 15g

2.13 Vegan Minestrone Soup

Ingredients

- Cubed bread: one cup

- Low-sodium vegetable broth: 3 cups

- Garlic: 5 cloves

- Leek: one cup (chopped)

- Olive oil: 3 tbsp.

- Carrots: one cup(chopped)

- Water: three cups

- Small pasta: one cup

- Kosher salt: 3/4 tsp.

- Beans: 15 ounces

- Baby kale: 3 cups

- Zucchini: 10 ounces (thinly sliced)

- Peas: 1 cup

- Ground pepper: half teaspoon

Instructions

- Let the oven Preheat oven to 350 F.

- Cook the garlic in two tablespoons of oil over medium heat in a medium skillet, stirring continuously for three minutes until the garlic is softened.

- Add bread; toss it to coat. Spread the combination uniformly on a baking dish. Bake, for ten minutes, until toasted.

- In the meanwhile, heat the leftover one tablespoon oil over medium flame in a big pan. Add the leek and carrots; simmer for five minutes, stirring frequently until softened.

- Add salt, broth, and water, cover it and bring to a simmer over a high flame.

- Add the pasta on low flame; cook uncovered for five minutes, stirring regularly. Then add zucchini, stirring regularly, for around five minutes, until the pasta is al dente.

- Stir in kale, beans, peas, and seasoning. Cook for around two minutes, stirring regularly until the kale is wilted.

- Pour the soup into six bowls, evenly garnish with the croutons.

Nutrition per serving: 267 calories| total fat 8.6g |carbohydrates 8.7g | protein 9.7g

2.14 Lemon Chicken Orzo Soup with Kale

Ingredients

- Chicken broth: 4 cups

- Chicken breasts: 4 cups (1-inch pieces)

- Dried oregano: 1 tsp.

- Olive oil: 2 tbsp.

- Salt: 1 and ¼ tsp.

- Diced onions: 2 cups

- One bay leaf

- Orzo pasta: 2/3 cup

- Diced celery: 1 cup

- Chopped kale: 4 cups

- Two minced cloves of Garlic

- Diced carrots: 1 cup

- One lemon juice and zest

- Black pepper: ¾ tsp.

Instructions

- Heat one tbsp. Of oil over medium flame in a big pot. Add the chicken, oregano (half teaspoon), salt, pepper. Cook for five minutes till light brown. move the chicken to the plate

- Add the remaining one spoonful of oil, carrots, onions, celery, and carrots in the same pot. Cook for five minutes until the vegetables are tender. Add the bay leaf, Garlic, and oregano (half teaspoon) cook for around 30 to 60 seconds,

- Add broth and let it boil over a high flame. Adding orzo. Then lower the heat for five minutes to let it simmer, cover, and let it cook. Add the chicken and kale and any leftover juices. Continue cooking for ten minutes until the orzo is soft and the chicken is cooked.

- Remove from flame. Throw away the bay leaf. Add lemon zest and lemon juice, 3/4 tsp, salt, and 1/4 tsp. of pepper.

- Serve right away.

Nutrition per serving: Calories 245|Net carbs 20g| protein 12 g|fat12 g| Cholesterol 17.6 mg| Sodium 214 mg| Potassium 220 mg| Phosphorus 187 mg| Calcium 29.2 mg| Fiber 2.4 g

2.15 Slow-Cooker Chicken & Chickpea Soup

Ingredients

- 8 cups bone-in, trimmed skin removed, chicken thighs,

- Dried chickpeas: 1 and a ½ cups (soaked overnight)

- Chopped red bell pepper: 1 and a half cup

- One large yellow onion, thinly sliced

- Tomato paste: 2 tablespoons

- 4 cups of water

- 4 cloves of garlic, minced

- One bay leaf

- Paprika: 4 teaspoons

- Ground cumin: 4 teaspoons

- ¼ of a teaspoon freshly ground black pepper

- ¼ of a cup halved pitted olives(oil-cured)

- Half of a teaspoon salt

- ¼ of a cup of chopped fresh parsley

- ¼ of a teaspoon cayenne pepper

Instructions

- Rinse and drain the chickpeas, put them in a large slow cooker, add four cups of water, chopped red pepper, bay leaf, tomato paste, and paprika cayenne, freshly ground black pepper, garlic, cumin.

- Mix well then, add the chicken.

- Cover it and cook on High for four hours or on low for at least 8 hours.

- Take out the chicken to a cutting surface and let it cool a little.

- Throw away the bay leaf. Then add olives, salt to the cooker and mix well.

- With forks, shred the chicken, set aside the bones. You would not need them.

- Add the shredded chicken into the soup.

- Garnish with cilantro and parsley.

- Serve hot.

Nutrition per serving: 446 calories| total fat 15.3g |carbohydrates 43g |protein 21.6g |Cholesterol 22.3 mg| Sodium 221 mg| Potassium 332 mg| Phosphorus 187 mg| Calcium 24 mg| Fiber 2.8 g

2.16 Ravioli & Vegetable Soup

Ingredients

- One package of fresh ravioli

- Red chopped bell pepper: one and a half cups

- Extra-virgin olive oil: 1 tablespoon

- Onion: 2 cups diced

- One can of 15 ounces' low sodium chicken broth or vegetable broth

- 1 and ½ cups of hot water

- Dried basil: 1 teaspoon

- 2 cups chopped zucchini

- 2 cloves of minced garlic

- Freshly ground black pepper, to taste

- 1/4 of a teaspoon crushed red pepper(optional)

Instructions

- Heat the oil over medium flame in a big saucepan or Dutch oven. Add the onion-pepper mixture, ground red pepper, garlic, and cook for one minute, stirring. Add water, red bell pepper, stock, basil over a high flame, let it boil.

- Add the ravioli and cook less than three minutes than the box instructs. Add the zucchini, let it boil again.

- Cook for about three minutes until the zucchini is soft, and adjust the taste by adding freshly ground black pepper

Nutrition per serving: 261 calories| total fat 8.3g | carbohydrates 32.6g |protein 10.6g

2.17 Hearty Chicken Soup

Ingredients

- Chicken broth, reduced-sodium: 4 cups

- 4 cups of chicken breasts, uncooked (skin and boneless), cubes

- 1 and a half cups celery

- Olive oil: 1 tablespoon

- Carrots: 1 cup, sliced

- 1 and a half cups onion, chopped
- Green beans: 1 cup, cut in 2 inch
- All-purpose white flour: 3 tablespoons
- Frozen green peas: 2 cups
- Dried basil: 2 teaspoons
- Nutmeg: 1/4 teaspoon
- Dried oregano: 1 teaspoon
- 1% low-fat milk: half cup
- Black pepper: 1/4 teaspoon
- Thyme: 1 teaspoon

Instructions

- In a skillet, cook the chicken for 5-6 minutes. Turn off the heat.
- In another pan, sauté celery and onion in heated olive oil.
- Add carrots, chicken pieces, flour, green beans, nutmeg, thyme, oregano, and basil— Cook for three minutes.
- Add milk; broth, let it boil.
- Add peas in. cook for five minutes.
- Add pepper and serve.

Nutrients per serving: Calories 131| Protein 14 g| Carbohydrates 12 g| Fat 3 g| Cholesterol 32 mg| Sodium 343 mg| Potassium 467 mg| phosphorus 171 mg| Calcium 67 mg| Fiber 2.8 g

2.18 Low Sodium Chicken Soup

Ingredients

- Onion: 1 tablespoon
- Mixed vegetables: 1 cup
- 4 cups of chicken breast cooked, shredded
- Four stalks of celery, chopped
- Carrots: 1 cup, chopped
- Butter: 1 tablespoon
- Chicken broth, low-sodium: 5 cups
- Fresh parsley: 2 tablespoons
- Seven and a half cups water
- Black pepper: 1/8 teaspoon

Instructions

- In a large pot, sauté onion in butter for five minutes.
- Add chicken broth and water let it boil.
- Add parsley, chicken, pepper, celery, cover it and let it simmer for half an hour.
- Add carrots, simmer for 20 minutes, then add frozen vegetables cook for another 20 minutes.
- Serve hot.

Nutrients per serving: Calories 97| Protein 13 g| Carbohydrates 5 g| Fat 3 g| Cholesterol 31 mg| Sodium 301 mg| Potassium 274 mg| Phosphorus 116 mg| Calcium 27 mg| Fiber 1.6 g

2.19 Barley & Beef Stew

Ingredients

- All-purpose white flour: 2 table-spoons

- Pearl barley: 1 cup, uncooked

- Black pepper: 1/4 teaspoon

- Half cup of onion, chopped

- Half teaspoon of salt

- 4 cups of stew meat, lean beef, cut into cubes

- Olive oil: 2 tablespoons

- 2 carrots, chopped

- One large stalk of celery, chopped

- One clove of garlic, minced

- Onion herb seasoning: 1 teaspoon

Instructions

- Soak barley in two cups of water for 60 minutes

- In a zip lock bag, add black pepper, stew meat, flour. Mix it well

- In a large pot, brown the meat in heated oil. Set it aside.

- Sauté garlic, onion, celery in meat residue for two minutes.

- Add 8 cups of water. Let it boil.

- Add bay leaf, salt, meat to the pot. Let it simmer.

- Drain barley, and add to the pot. Cover it let it cook for one hour. Stir occasionally.

- After one hour, add herb seasoning, carrots. Let it simmer for 60 minutes.

- Add more water if needed.

Nutrients per serving: Calories 246| Protein 22 g| Carbohydrates 21 g| Fat 8 g| Cholesterol 51 mg| Sodium 222 mg| Potassium 369 mg| phosphorus 175 mg| Calcium 30 mg| Fiber 6.3 g

2.20 Beef Stew with Carrots & Mushrooms

Ingredients

- Beef broth, low-sodium: 4 cups

- Onion chopped: 2 cups

- 3 cloves of garlic, minced

- Carrots, 2 cups diced

- Potato: 1 cup(leached)

- Stew meat, lean beef: 2 pounds

- Olive oil: 2 tablespoons

- Dry red wine: 1 cup

- Shitake mushrooms: 1 cup, sliced

- Dried thyme: half tablespoon

- All-purpose white flour: 1/3 cup

- One bay leaf

- Half teaspoon black pepper

- Herb seasoning: 3/4 teaspoon

Instructions

- In a Dutch oven, over medium flame, heat 2 tsp. of olive oil

- Sauté onion, add thyme, mushrooms cook for five minutes. Add garlic and cook for one minute.

- Add red wine and stir.

- Coat the beef in flour. In a large pan, over medium flame, heat two teaspoons of oil.

- Brown the beef and add herb seasoning. Add beef into mushroom mix.

- Add the broth and bay leaf. Let it boil.

- Cover it, turn the heat low, simmer for one hour.

- Add carrot, potatoes with beef. Simmer uncovered for 1 hour, stir as the soup thickens.

- Add black pepper. Take out the bay leaf and serve.

Nutrients per serving: Calories 282| Protein 33 g| Carbohydrates 15 g| Fat 10 g| Cholesterol 88 mg| Sodium 110 mg| Potassium 534 mg| Phosphorus 252 mg| Calcium 39 mg| Fiber 2.5 g|

2.21 Mediterranean Soup Jar

Ingredients

- Red pepper flakes: 1/8 teaspoon

- Black olives, reduced-sodium: 3 large

- Half cup of bell pepper & onion strips

- Half tablespoon of garlic & herb seasoning

- Canned chickpeas, no salt added: 1/3 cup

- Half teaspoon of black pepper

- Extra virgin olive oil: 1 teaspoon

- Half cup of coleslaw mix

- Cheese: 1 tablespoon

Instructions

- Wash the chickpeas and Slice the olives.

- Layer all ingredients in a big jar.

- Keep in Refrigerate until ready to serve.

- Take out from the fridge at least 15 minutes before serving.

- Add a half cup and a little more boiling water to the jar and shake the jar with a closed lid. Let it rest for two minutes. Then open and serve.

Nutrients per serving: Calories 222| Protein 7 g| Carbohydrates 26 g| Fat 10 g| Cholesterol 8 mg| Sodium 184 mg| Potassium 396 mg| Phosphorus 118 mg| Calcium 91 mg| Fiber 6.0 g

2.22 Green Chili Stew

Ingredients

- 1.75 cups of chicken broth, low-sodium

- Six flour tortillas

- Half cup of all-purpose flour

- One teaspoon of black pepper

- 4 cups of lean pork chops

- One cup of canned green chili peppers

- Olive oil: 1 tablespoon

- One tablespoon of garlic powder

- Iceberg lettuce: 3/4 cup

- One clove of garlic

- Cilantro: 1/4 cup

Instructions

- In a zip lock bag, add garlic powder, black pepper, and flour and mix. Add pork (bite sizes) pieces in the bag and coat well

- In a pot, brown the pork in olive oil.

- In a slow cooker, add minced garlic, chicken broth, browned pork, diced chili peppers—Cook for ten hours on low.

- Add ¾ cup stew on tortilla and serve with cilantro and lettuce. Or eat as it is.

Nutrients per serving: Calories 420| Protein 25 g| Carbohydrates 44 g| Fat 16 g| Cholesterol 45 mg| Sodium 552 mg| Potassium 454 mg| Phosphorus 323 mg| Calcium 90 mg| fiber 3.2 g

2.23 Kidney-Friendly Vegetable Soup

Ingredients

- Olive oil: 1 tablespoon

- 1 medium onion

- 2 sticks celery

- 2 large cloves of garlic

- Six large carrots

- One cube of chicken or vegetable low sodium

- 1 medium turnip

- Water: 1 and 1.2 l

- Fresh thyme

- One bay leaf

- Black pepper

Instructions

- Chop all the vegetables

- In a pot, add carrots and turnip, add water four times of their volume

- Let it boil until tender

- in a heavy-based pan, heat the olive oil.

- Add the celery, onion, and garlic—Cook for a few minutes.

- Cover it and cook on low heat for 15 minutes. Make sure it is not burning.

- After 15 minutes, add boiled turnip and carrots. Dissolve cube in water.

- Pour the stock into the vegetable mix, add thyme and bay leaf, pepper

- Let it boil and simmer for half an hour, take out the bay leaf

- Puree the soup in a blender. Add more water if too thick

Nutrition per serving: Calories: 42kcal| Carbohydrate Content: 5.7g|Fat Content: 1.6g|Protein Content: 1g|Salt: 0.1g|Sugar Content: 4.6g|Potassium: 3.3mg|Phosphate: 23mg

2.24 Yucatan Lime Soup

Ingredients

- Eight cloves of garlic, minced

- Chicken breast: 1 and a half cups cooked, shredded
- Two serrano chili peppers, chopped
- Chicken broth, low-sodium: 4 cups
- One small tomato
- Cilantro: 1/4 cup, chopped
- Half cup of onion, diced
- Two tortillas, cut into strips
- Olive oil: 1 tablespoon
- 1/4 teaspoon of salt
- Black pepper
- 1 bay leaf
- Lime juice: 1/4 cup

Instructions

- Let the oven preheat to 400° F.
- place tortilla strips on a baking tray and spray with oil. Bake for three minutes or till slightly toasted. Take out from the oven and set it aside.
- In a pot, sauté chili, garlic, and onion in olive oil, till translucent
- Add salt, chicken, tomato, bay leaf, and chicken. Simmer for ten minutes.
- Add black pepper, cilantro, lime juice.
- Serve with toasted strips.

Nutrients per serving: Calories 214| Protein 20 g| Carbohydrates 12 g| Fat 10 g| Cholesterol 32 mg| Sodium 246 mg| Potassium 355 mg| Phosphorus 176 mg|Calcium 47 mg| Fiber 1.6 g

2.25 Sausage Egg Soup

Ingredients

- 4 egg whites
- 2 cups of ground beef
- Half teaspoon of ground sage
- Olive oil: 2 tablespoons
- Half teaspoon of dried basil
- Day-old 4 slices bread
- Half teaspoon of black pepper
- Herb seasoning: 1 tablespoon
- Half teaspoon of garlic powder
- Grated parmesan cheese: 2 tablespoons
- Two cloves of garlic
- Chicken broth, low-sodium: 3 cups
- 1 and a half cups water
- Fresh parsley: 4 tablespoons

Instructions

- Let the oven preheat to 375° F.
- In a bowl, mix black pepper, ground beef, garlic powder, sage, and basil. Set it aside
- Cut bread into cubes and add herb seasoning, olive oil. Bake for 8 minutes or until golden brown. Set aside.
- Fry the sausage (beef mix) until it's done. Take out from the pan and drain.

- Sauté the garlic in 2 tbsp. Of drippings. Add parsley, water, broth

- Cover it and let it boil, simmer for ten minutes.

- Turn the heat to low. Gently add egg whites.

- Serve with croutons and cheese.

Nutrients per serving: Calories 335| Protein 26 g| Carbohydrates 15 g| Fat 19 g| Cholesterol 250 mg| Sodium 374 mg| potassium 392 mg| Phosphorus 268 mg| Calcium 118 mg| Fiber 0.9 g

2.26 Chicken Corn Soup

Ingredients

- Water: 14 cups

- 4 pound of roasting chicken

- Dried parsley: 1 tablespoon

- Half cups and a little more un-cooked flat noodles

- 2 cans of unsalted corn

- Black pepper: 1/4 teaspoon

Instructions

- In a pot, cook chicken in 8 cups of water. Reserve the broth and cooked chicken separately.

- Cook the noodles as per instructions, without salt. Set it aside.

- Take the fat out from chicken broth. Chop the chicken into pieces.

- In a big pot, add 6 cups of broth, 6 cups of water, chopped chicken.

- Add parsley, corns, pepper, cooked noodles. Let it simmer and then serve

Nutrients per serving: Calories 222| Protein 25 g| Carbohydrates 17 g| Fat 6 g| Cholesterol 67 mg| Sodium 240 mg| Potassium 303 mg| Phosphorus 212 mg| Calcium 21 mg| Fiber 1.4 g

2.27 Moroccan Chicken Soup

Ingredients

- Spaghetti pasta: 2 cups

- 4 cups of skinless chicken legs,

- One cup of zucchini

- Cilantro: 1 tablespoon

- Seven and a half cups of water

- Half teaspoon of cumin

- Half teaspoon of turmeric

- Couscous: 1 cup, dry

- Chickpeas: 1/3 cup

- Black pepper: 1 teaspoon

- Half teaspoon of salt

Instructions

- In a pot, add chicken legs with six cups of water, simmer for almost one hour or until cooked.

- Add spaghetti and chickpeas to the soup and simmer for 15 minutes.

- Add chopped cilantro, zucchini, spices to the soup. Cook for another 15 minutes.

- Prepare couscous as you like. Serve with hot soup.

Nutrients per serving: Calories 224| Protein 18 g| Carbohydrates 29 g| Fat 4 g| Cholesterol 42 mg| Sodium 313 mg| potassium 296 mg| Phosphorus 148 mg| calcium 42 mg| Fiber 3.0 g

2.28 Italian Wedding Soup

Ingredients

- 1 cup uncooked pasta
- 4 cups of ground beef (extra-lean)
- Dried bread crumbs: 1/4 cup
- Grated cheese: 2 tablespoons
- Cooked chicken: 2 cups, diced
- 2 large egg whites
- Dried basil: 1 teaspoon
- Fresh kale leaves: 1 cup
- Carrots: 3/4 cup, diced
- Low-sodium chicken broth: 10 cups
- Chopped onion: 3 tablespoons

Instructions

- In a bowl, add eggs, cheese, onion, beef, basil, bread crumbs. mix well
- Make small meatballs.
- In a pot, add chicken broth, heat it. Add pasta, kale, meatballs, carrots.
- Let it slow boil for ten minutes, then turn the heat down low.
- Add chicken. Make sure meats balls and pasta is cooked before serving.

Nutrients per serving: Calories 165| Protein 21 g| Carbohydrates 11 g| Fat 6 g| Cholesterol 73 mg| Sodium 276 mg| Potassium 360 mg| phosphorus 176 mg| Calcium 42 mg| Fiber 1.0 g

2.29 Vegan Chickpeas & Mushroom Soup

Ingredients

- Half onion chopped
- Dried Italian seasoning: 1 tablespoon
- 2 cloves garlic minced
- 2 cups of sliced mushrooms
- 1 can of chickpeas
- Olive oil: 1 tbsp.
- Salt & pepper to taste
- Vegetable broth: 3 cups
- Dried rosemary: 1 teaspoon
- Pinch, hot pepper flakes

Instructions

- In a pan, sauté onion, garlic in olive oil until slightly brown.
- Add mushrooms after a minute or two, add chickpeas and spices. Add salt and pepper.
- Cook for 3 to 5 minutes, add broth and let it boil. Add chili flakes, and let it simmer for half an hour.
- Then blend it in a blender. Pour back in pot heat it through.

Nutrition per serving: Calories: 197kcal | Carbohydrates: 31g | Protein:

11g | Fat: 4g | Sodium: 790mg | Potassium: 879mg | Fiber: 7g | Sugar: 4g | Vitamin A: 415IU | Vitamin C: 3.9mg | Calcium: 107mg | Iron: 4.2mg

2.30 Carrot Soup

Ingredients

- 1 cup carrot, shredded
- 1 teaspoon curry paste
- 1 tablespoon olive oil
- 1 yellow onion, diced
- ½ teaspoon chili flakes
- 1 tablespoon lemon juice
- 2 cups low-sodium chicken broth

Instructions

- Heat olive oil in the saucepan and add the onion. Cook it until light brown.
- Add grated carrot, curry paste, chili flakes, and chicken broth.
- Close the lid and cook the soup for 25 minutes.
- Then blend it with the help of the immersion blender until smooth.
- Add lemon juice and cook the soup for 5 minutes more.

Nutrition per serving: 92 calories|2.2g protein|8.3g carbohydrates|5.7g fat|1.7g fiber| 0mg cholesterol|74mg sodium, |178mg potassium.

2.31 Pasta Soup

Ingredients

- 2 oz. whole-grain pasta
- ½ cup corn kernels
- 1 oz. carrot, shredded
- 3 oz. celery stalk, chopped
- 2 cups low-sodium chicken stock
- 1 teaspoon ground black pepper

Instructions

- Bring the chicken stock to boil and add shredded carrot and celery stalk. Simmer the liquid for 5 minutes.
- After this, add corn kernels, ground black pepper, and pasta. Mix the soup well.
- Simmer it on the medium heat for 8 minutes.

Nutrition per serving: Calories: 140 kcal| Protein: 4 g| Carbohydrates: 21 g| Dietary Fiber: 2 g| Phosphorus: 79 mg| Potassium: 224 mg|Sodium: 52 mg

2.32 Chicken & Rice Soup

Ingredients

- Two chicken breasts, cubed cooked, boneless and skinless
- 3 cup chopped mixed vegetables
- Celery: 1 cup, diced
- Black pepper
- Baby carrot: 1 cup chopped
- Onion: 1 cup, diced
- Extra virgin oil: 2 tbsp.
- Four thyme sprigs
- Lime juice: 2 tbsp.

- One bay leaf
- Instant white rice: ¾ cup uncooked
- Vegetable/chicken broth, no salt added: 10 cups

Instructions

- In a pot, in olive oil, sauté celery, carrots, and onion. Until tender.
- Add fresh thyme, pepper, stock, bay leaf, and rice. Let it boil.
- Lower the heat and let it simmer for 12-15 minutes
- Add cooked chicken. Let it Simmer for ten minutes.
- Take out bay leaf, add lime juice serve hot

Nutrient per serving: Calories: 160 g| Protein: 14 g| Carbohydrates: 19 g| Fiber: 2 g| Total Fat: 3 g| Sodium: 221 mg| Phosphorus: 90 mg| Potassium: 251 mg|

2.33 Beef Stew

Ingredients

- Five chopped carrots
- stew meat, Lean beef: 8 cups
- 3 celery stalks, diced
- One onion, diced
- 3 cloves of minced garlic
- Sliced mushrooms: 1 cup
- One potato diced (leached)
- Salt-free table seasoning: 1 teaspoon

- One can of beef broth, low sodium
- All-purpose flour: 5 tablespoons
- Dry red wine: 1 cup
- Olive oil: 2 tablespoons

Instructions

- Coat the beef in seasoning and flour mix. In a pot, in olive oil, brown the beef, take the meat out, add all vegetables, do not add carrots, and cook until onions are translucent.
- Lower the heat, add in the red wine. Let it simmer for five minutes, add in the cooked beef.
- Add broth, let it boil. Lower the heat, let it simmer, covered, for 60 minutes. Add in the carrots and potatoes.
- Let it Simmer uncovered for 60 minutes. Add spices, salt-free seasonings, and herbs to your taste.

Nutrient per serving: Calories: 193 g| Protein: 14.4 g| Carbohydrates: 18.2 g| Fiber: 2 g| Total Fat: 3.4 g| Sodium: 227 mg| Phosphorus: 111 mg| Potassium: 198 mg|

2.34 Tuscan Vegetable Soup

Ingredients

- Chicken broth, low sodium: 8 cups
- Olive oil: 1 tablespoon
- Thyme: 1 and a half teaspoons, dried

- Garlic: 3 teaspoons, minced
- Onion: 1 and a half cups, finely chopped
- Green cabbage: 4 cups, roughly chopped
- 1 can chickpeas: 15 ounce
- Celery: 2 cups, sliced
- Baby carrots: 2 cups, diced
- One cup of bell pepper
- Parmesan cheese: 1 tablespoon shredded
- Half cup basil, chopped fresh
- Zucchini: 3 cups, sliced

Instructions

- In a pot, sauté garlic, onion, and thyme for 3 to 5 minutes
- Add in the chickpeas, bell peppers, cabbage, carrots, celery, sauté for ten minutes
- Add in zucchini, chicken broth, basil, let it boil.
- Then lower the heat, let it simmer, cover it saucepan, let it simmer for 40 minutes or more
- Add cheese on top while serving.

Nutritional per serving: Calories 137| protein 7.6 g| Carbohydrates 24 g| Dietary fiber 5.3 g| fat 2.7 g| Saturated fat0.6 g| cholesterol 0.3 mg| Sodium 272 mg| Calcium79.6 mg| Iron 2.1 mg| Potassium 718 mg

2.35 Healthy Chicken Wild Rice Soup

Ingredients

- Chicken broth or water: 9 cups
- 6 cups of chicken pieces
- 2 cloves of minced garlic
- 2 cups sliced mushrooms
- Two carrots, roughly chopped
- Cauliflower: one and a half cups
- 3 celery stalks, chopped
- One large onion, finely diced
- Almond milk: 2 cups
- Wild rice: 1 and a half cups
- Mustard: 1 tbsp.
- Garlic powder: 2 tsp
- Ground black pepper, to taste
- Half tsp dried thyme
- 2 tsp of salt

Instructions

- In a slow cooker, add garlic, chicken, celery, onion, carrots, mushrooms, cauliflower, pepper, wild rice, salt, water, and thyme. Cover it and cook for 8-10 hours on Low or for 5-6 hours on High.
- Take chicken out and shred it. in the slow cooker, add garlic powder, milk, and mustard
- Blend the soup and return to the pot.

- Add the shredded chicken, serve hot

Nutrition per serving: Calories 251 kcal | Sodium 123 mg| Protein 13.2 g| Potassium 292 mg| phosphorus 131 mg| Calcium 25.4 mg| Fat 8.9 g| | Carbohydrates 8.6 g

2.36 Beef & Vegetable Soup

Ingredients

- Carrots: ½ cup, diced
- 4 cups of beef stew
- Sliced onions: 1 cup
- Basil: ½ tsp
- Green peas: ½ cup
- 3 ½ cup of water
- Black pepper: 1 tsp
- Corn: ½ cup
- Okra: ½ cup
- Thyme: ½ tsp

Instructions

- In a pot, add black pepper, beef stew, water, onions, thyme, and basil
- Cook for 45 minutes.
- Add all vegetables let it simmer on low heat till meat is tender. Enjoy.

Nutrition per serving: Calories 190 kcal | Sodium 56 mg| Protein 11 g| Potassium 291 mg| phosphorus 121 mg| Calcium 31 mg| Fat 13 g| Water 130 g| Carbohydrates 7 g

2.37 Healing Cauliflower Holiday Soup

Ingredients

- Vegetable broth, low sodium: 4 cups
- Olive oil: 1 tablespoon
- 3 cloves of minced garlic
- 6 cups of cauliflower, chopped
- Leeks sliced: 2 cups
- Nutmeg: 3/4 teaspoon
- Red pepper flakes: half teaspoon
- Half teaspoon pepper
- 2 cups of water
- Half teaspoon salt
- 1/4 cup cashews

Instructions

- In a pot, sauté garlic, leeks, cook for about two minutes
- Add spices and cauliflower, sauté for five minutes.
- Add the broth, water, let it boil, then let it simmer, covered, for at least 20 minutes. Longer if you need it.
- Add cashews, and blend the soup. Add water if too thick
- Transfer soup back in the pot. Season and taste with pepper and salt.

Nutrition per serving: Calories: 187 kcal | Carbohydrates: 21.5 g | Protein:

10g | Fat: 5g | Sodium: 645 mg | Potassium: 345 mg | Fiber: 4.5 g | Sugar: 5g | Calcium: 65 mg | Iron: 3.8mg

2.38 Vegetarian Cabbage Soup

Ingredients

- 2 cloves of minced garlic
- 4 cups of cabbage, shredded
- 2 cups of cauliflower, cut into cubes
- One large onion, chopped
- Vegetable broth, low sodium: 4 cups
- 2 big carrots, cut into cubes
- Olive oil: 1 tbsp.
- 2 cups of diced bell pepper
- 2 stalks of sliced celery
- Two pinches of chili flakes
- 3-4 bay leaves
- Paprika: 1 tsp
- Salt & pepper, to taste

Instructions

- In a pot, sauté celery, paprika, onion, bay leaves, carrots, chili flakes, garlic in hot olive oil.
- Cook for five minutes.
- Add shredded cabbage and keep stirring for one minute.
- Add red peppers, cauliflower florets, broth, and a pinch of salt.
- Increase the heat and let it boil, then cover it, and let it simmer for 25 minutes.

- Then, remove the bay leaves.
- Blend the soup in the blender. Return soup to the pot, season with salt and pepper.

Nutrition per serving: Calories: 146kcal | Carbohydrates: 25g | Protein: 5g | Fat: 4g | Saturated Fat: 1g | Sodium: 117mg | Potassium: 846mg | Fiber: 9g | Sugar: 12g | Calcium: 125mg | Iron: 2mg

2.39 Slow Cooker Cabbage Soup

Ingredients

- Two cloves of minced garlic
- Carrots: 1 cup, diced
- One onion diced
- Cabbage: 4 cups, chopped
- Green beans: 1 cup trimmed into one-inch pieces
- 2 celery stalks diced
- 2 bell peppers diced
- Tomato paste: 2 tablespoons
- 2 bay leaves
- Fresh kale: 2 cups roughly chopped
- Low sodium stock vegetable: 6 cups
- Italian seasoning: 1 and a half tsp.
- Pepper
- Basil: 1 tablespoon
- Parsley: 1 tablespoon

Instructions

- In a pot, add vegetables. Add tomato paste, Italian seasoning, broth, pepper, bay leaves. Mix well

- Cook on high for five hours or slow on 8 hours in a slow cooker.

- After its cooked, add basil, parsley, kale, and cook for five minutes and serve.

Nutrition per serving: Calories: 40|Carbohydrates: 6g| Protein: 2g|Sodium: 64mg| Potassium: 158mg| Fiber: 1g| Sugar: 2g| Vitamin A: 2230IU| Vitamin C: 32.5mg| Calcium: 28mg|Iron: 0.7mg

2.40 Healthy Mushroom Soup

Ingredients

- Vegetable broth: 2 cups

- 4 cups of mushrooms, roughly chopped

- 3 garlic cloves, minced

- Soya sauce, low sodium: 1 tbsp.

- Olive oil: 2 tbsp.

- One onion, chopped

- Thyme leaves: half tsp

- All-purpose flour: 1/4 cup

- Soy milk: 1 cup

- Salt & black pepper to taste

Instructions

- In a large pot, sauté garlic, onions in olive oil for 3 minutes.

- Add thyme, mushrooms, salt, pepper. Cook until the mushroom starts to turn brown for five minutes. Take out three tbsp. of mushroom and set them aside

- Add in the one tbsp. of oil, flour cook for half a minute.

- Now add broth and mix well. Let the mixture boil. Then let it simmer and lower the heat. Add milk

- Simmer again, often stirring, for 15-20 minutes.

- Add the soya sauce and stir for one minute

- Add salt if required.

- Serve with sautéed mushrooms on top.

Nutrition per serving: Calories: 213kcal | Carbohydrates: 22g | Protein: 10g | Fat: 11g | Saturated Fat: 2g | Cholesterol: 4mg | Sodium: 379mg | Potassium: 656mg | Fiber: 3g | Sugar: 9g | Calcium: 110mg | Iron: 1mg

2.41 Green Beans Soup

Ingredients

- ½ onion, diced

- 1/3 cup green beans, soaked

- 3 cups of water

- ½ sweet pepper, chopped

- 2 potatoes, chopped

- One tablespoon fresh cilantro, chopped

- 1 teaspoon chili flakes

Instructions

- In the saucepan, put all the ingredients and close the lid.
- On medium heat, cook the soup for 40 minutes or until the ingredients are all tender
- Serve.

Nutrients Per serving: 87 calories|2.3g protein|19.8g carbohydrates| 0.2g fat| 3.4g fiber|0mg cholesterol|13 mg sodium| 132 mg potassium.

2.42 Pureed Broccoli Soup

Ingredients

- 1tbsp. unsalted Butter
- Olive Oil: 1tbsp.
- Chicken Broth low-sodium 4cups
- Onion: one (chopped).
- 2 cloves of minced garlic
- Fresh Thyme
- Broccoli 8 cups chopped
- Celery stalk: one, chopped
- Water 2cups
- Non-dairy creamer half cup, optional
- Freshly Ground Pepper to taste
- Salt: ½ tsp

Instructions

- In a large pot, sauté celery, onion in butter until tender for 5-6 minutes

- Add thyme and garlic, cook for ten seconds.
- Add in broccoli. Add broth and water, let it simmer for 8 minutes.
- Blend the soup in a blender. Add creamer and black pepper

Nutrition Per Serving: Calories 69| protein 4g.| Carbohydrate 7g.|Total Fat 4g.| Cholesterol 4mg.| Potassium 230mg.| Sodium 258mg.| Phosphorus 45mg.|

2.43 Zucchini Curry Soup Recipe

Ingredients

- Extra virgin olive oil: 2 tbsp.
- A large onion
- Red curry powder: 2 tbsp.
- Chicken broth: 3 cups
- Plain Greek yogurt
- Five large zucchini
- Salt and pepper, to taste

Instructions

- Cut zucchini, onion into pieces.
- In a pan, sauté vegetables, with curry, pepper, and salt in olive oil, until tender
- Add the broth. Cover it and let it cook for 20 minutes.
- Blend the soup in a blender till smooth.
- Taste salt and pepper and adjust.

- Garnish with tablespoon plain Greek yogurt

Nutrition per serving: Calories: 89kcal | Carbohydrates: 8g | Protein: 2g | Fat: 5g | Saturated Fat: 0g | Cholesterol: 0mg | Sodium: 445mg | Potassium: 579mg | Fiber: 2g | Sugar: 4g | Vitamin A: 345IU | Vitamin C: 39mg | Calcium: 47mg | Iron: 1.5mg

2.44 Butternut Squash & Apple Soup

Ingredients

- 2 red apples diced
- one peeled butternut squash, cut into cubes
- one fennel bulb nicely chopped
- 4 – 5 cloves of garlic cloves
- Olive oil: 1/4 cup
- Rosemary: 1 tablespoon
- One white onion chopped
- Vegetable broth: 4 cups
- Ground cinnamon: half teaspoon
- Dried thyme: 1 teaspoon
- Nutmeg: 1/4 teaspoon
- Salt & pepper
- Water as needed
- Ginger: 1/4 teaspoon

Instructions

- Let the oven preheat to 400 F.
- Mix all the spices and oil. Pour over onion, squash, garlic, fennel, and apples. Mix it well and roast the vegetables for 30 to 40 minutes. Shake vegetables half-way, so they do not burn.
- Add the roasted vegetables to the pot, add broth and let it boil.
- Turn down the heat and let it simmer for 10-12 minutes, or until everything is tender.
- Blend the soup, in a blender, until creamy and smooth
- Add water as required. Serve warm

Nutrition per serving: Calories: 200kcal | Carbohydrates: 30g | Protein: 2g | Fat: 9g | Saturated Fat: 1g | Sodium: 412 mg | Potassium: 423 mg | Fiber: 5g | Sugar: 11g | Calcium: 99mg | Iron: 1.7mg

2.45 Lemon & Garlic Wild Rice Soup

Ingredients

- Italian seasoning, low sodium: 1 tablespoon
- Olive oil: 1 tablespoon
- Lemon zest: 1 tablespoon
- Chopped carrots: 1 cup
- Sliced celery: 1 cup
- Five garlic of minced cloves
- Half cup white onion
- Lemon juice: 1/4 cup
- Salt & pepper
- Half cup of wild rice
- Almond milk: 1 cup

- Fresh kale: 1 cup
- Vegetable broth, low sodium: 4 cups

Instructions

- In a large pot, sauté carrots, garlic, onion, celery, in olive oil, until tender for five minutes. Add all the seasonings, zest, and cook for three minutes.
- Add in the rice, vegetable broth and let it boil. Cover it and let it simmer until rice has cooked for half an hour or more.
- Add in the milk, lemon juice, kale once the rice is cooked. Cook until kale is wilted.
- Serve immediately.

Nutrition per serving: Calories: 162kcal | Carbohydrates: 27g | Protein: 4g | Fat: 4g | Sodium: 245 mg | Potassium: 370mg | Fiber: 4g | Sugar: 5g | Calcium: 139mg | Iron: 1.3mg

2.46 Gingered Carrot Bisque

Ingredients

- Diced celery: half cup
- Olive oil: 1 tablespoon
- One-piece (1-1/2) of ginger, finely diced
- Vegetable broth: 4 cups
- Diced onion: 3/4 cup
- Salt
- No salt curry powder: 1 and 1/2 teaspoons

- No salt cashew cream: 1/3 cup, optional
- One carrot diced

Instructions

- In a pot, sauté ginger, celery, and onion until translucent.
- Add in curry powder, broth, potato, carrots, let it boil.
- Lower the heat and let it simmer. Stir occasionally, for 25 minutes.
- Blend the soup in a blender. Pour it back into the pot.
- Cook on low heat until heated through.
- Add in the cashew cream if you want.
- Serve hot.

Nutrition per serving: Calories: 261 kcal | Carbohydrates: 35g | Protein: 10g | Fat: 22g | Saturated Fat: 3g | Sodium: 256 mg | Potassium: 213mg | Fiber: 5g | Sugar: 5 g | Calcium: 29.9 mg | Iron: 3.8mg

2.47 Roasted Garlic Cauliflower Chowder

Ingredients

- Vegetable broth, low sodium: 2 cups
- Cashews soaked: half cup
- One small potato(leached) chopped
- One garlic bulb

- One head of cauliflower, cut into florets
- Oil: 2 tablespoons
- Half cup of garlic hummus, low sodium
- Water: 2 cups
- Miso paste: 2 teaspoons
- Half cup cooked quinoa
- Salt and pepper to taste

Instructions

- Let the oven preheat to 425°F.
- Put cauliflower and potato, cut the garlic bulb in two-three pieces but wrap in foil, on a baking tray. Add one tbsp. of oil, add pepper and salt
- Roast for 20 to 25 minutes till cauliflower starts to brown, and the potatoes become soft. Check the garlic after 15 minutes. It should not be burning.
- Cook the vegetables for 5-10 minutes, then blend it. Take the skin of garlic and mix it also.
- Add cashew to a blender, with quinoa and hummus. Add in miso, liquids, pepper, and salt. Blend on high until creamy.
- Adjust seasoning to your taste.

Nutrition per serving: Calories: 284kcal | Carbohydrates: 25g | Protein: 9g | Fat: 17g | Saturated Fat: 2g | Sodium: 794mg | Potassium: 536mg | Fiber: 5g | Sugar: 2g| Calcium: 47mg | Iron: 4.1mg

2.48 Golden Soup

Ingredients

- Cauliflower, 5 cups of florets
- Oil: 2 tablespoons olive
- Half onion, chopped
- 2 cloves of garlic, minced
- Water: 7–8 cups
- Turmeric: 1 tablespoon
- One tsp. Of salt
- Lemon juice

Instructions

- In a pot, sauté garlic, turmeric, onion, cauliflower in oil for ten minutes.
- Add water and salt let it simmer. Transfer the soup to a blender till it becomes creamy.
- Take the blended soup into the pot again. Add more water if required. Season with salt if needed. Add lemon juice.

Nutrition Per Serving: Calories 180| Total Fat 13.3g| Cholesterol 0mg| Sodium 213.3mg| Total Carbohydrate 13.2g| Dietary Fiber 3.1g|sugars 3.6g| Protein 5.7g

2.49 Anti-Inflammatory Thai Pumpkin Soup

Ingredients

- 4 cloves of sliced garlic
- Pumpkin: 600 g
- Soy milk: ½ cup

- Olive oil: 1 tablespoon
- Vegetable stock: 3 cups
- Lemongrass: 1 tablespoon (white part), diced
- Two shredded kaffir lime leaves
- One turmeric sliced
- Coriander seeds: 1 teaspoon
- One small red chili de-seeded, thinly sliced
- Cumin seeds: 1 teaspoon
- One onion, diced
- Black pepper
- One-inch ginger minced

Instructions

- Let the oven preheat to 350 F. Add baking paper on a tray.
- Chop the peeled pumpkin, coat with soy milk, and roast until golden.
- In a pot, heat oil, sauté onion till golden, add coriander seeds, cumin
- Cook for a few minutes
- Add garlic, lemongrass, chili, ginger, kaffir leaves, turmeric, cook for another minute. Do not overcook
- Add broth and pumpkin, cover it and let it boil. Let it simmer for t10 minutes. Add milk, increase the heat.
- Cook for 5-10 minutes.

Nutrition per serving: Calories: 349kcal | Carbohydrates: 35g | Protein: 11g | Fat: 21g | Saturated Fat: 17g | Sodium: 225mg | Fiber: 3g | Sugar: 11g | Calcium: 130mg | Iron: 5.8mg

2.50 Turkey Vegetable Soup

Ingredients

- Two medium onions, diced
- 2 tablespoons of flour
- Unsalted butter: 1/4 cup
- Low-sodium curry powder: 1 and a half teaspoons
- Lean ground turkey: 2 pounds, cooked
- Half cup of carrots, diced
- Low-sodium chicken broth
- Half cup celery, diced
- Parsley: 2 tablespoons
- Half teaspoon sage, diced
- One and a half cups of soy milk
- Frozen chopped kale: 1 and ¼ cups
- 1 cup potatoes, leached and diced
- Black Pepper

Instructions

- In the pot, melt butter over medium flame
- Sauté onions cook until translucent, for ten minutes
- Stir in curry powder and flour, cook for 2-3 minutes

- Add potatoes, broth, parsley, carrots, sage, and celery
- Let it boil. Turn the heat low. cover it and simmer for ten minutes
- Add kale, turkey, and milk
- Cover it and simmer until all heated through
- Add black pepper.

Nutrition per serving: Calories 245| Fat 13.8 g| Carbohydrates 8 g| protein 24 g| Dietary Fiber 1.5 g| Calcium 49 mg| Phosphorous 270 mg| Sodium 125 mg| Potassium 498 mg

2.51 Cauliflower Soup

Ingredients

- Margarine: 1 Tbsp.
- Three cups of water
- Chicken bouillon, low-sodium: 1/4 cube
- Low-fat mayonnaise: 1 Tbsp.
- Half onion, diced
- 1/4 cup celery, diced
- 1 cup of cauliflower, diced
- Three baby carrots, sliced
- 1 Tbsp. Flour
- Pepper: 1/4 tsp.
- Dried basil: 1/8 tsp
- Cream cheese: 3 Tbsp.
- Half tsp. of salt
- 2 minced garlic

Instructions

- In a pot, add the bouillon cube, water, celery, onion, and carrots. Let it boil over low heat.
- Add cream cheese, salt, mayonnaise, pepper, herbs, and one tbsp. of margarine.
- Add cauliflower to soup and cook for five minutes.
- Add cornstarch to water and add in the soup. Stir until thickens, and serve

Nutrition per serving: Calories: 57 | protein 2 g |Sodium 212 mg | Phosphorus 32 mg| Calcium 36 mg | Potassium 156 mg|

Chapter 3: Kidney-Friendly Pasta Recipes

3.1 Pasta Primavera

Ingredients

- All-purpose white flour: 2 tablespoons
- One and a half cup of uncooked pasta,
- 2 cups of chicken broth, low-sodium
- Non-dairy creamer: 1/4 cup
- One and a half cup of frozen mixed vegetables
- Grated Parmesan cheese: 1/4 cup

Instructions

- Cook vegetables and pasta separately, as per instruction on boxes. Set them aside.

- In a pot, add chicken broth on low flame

- Add flour to the chicken broth keep whisking, so lumps will not form

- Add garlic powder, creamer, and mix.

- Let it simmer for 5 -10 minutes or until it thickens.

- Stir sometimes, while it is simmering.

- Add cooked pasta and vegetable and cook till all heated through.

- Sprinkle with cheese.

Nutrients per serving: Calories 273|Protein 13 g| Carbohydrates 48 g| Fat 3 g| Cholesterol 6 mg| sodium 115 mg| Potassium 251 mg| Phosphorus 154 mg| Calcium 93 mg| Fiber 4.5 g

3.2 The Best Pasta Ever

Ingredients

- 4 oz. of uncooked Spaghetti Noodles

- Extra-virgin olive oil: 2 Tbsp.

- Half small minced Onion

- Dried Cranberries: 1/4 cup

- Kale: 4 cups

- Crumbled Feta Cheese: 2 Tbsp.

- Six cloves of sliced Garlic

- Water: 1/4 cup

Instructions

- In a skillet, sauté garlic in olive oil, over medium flame, until slices are lightly golden brown. Take out the slices and set it aside.

- Lower the heat, add onion, add pepper and salt for three minutes

- Add kale; cranberries add more pepper, salt if required. Add water, cover it, and let it cook for five minutes.

- Cook spaghetti as per instructions.

- Add spaghetti to the skillet, then toss everything. Add 1/4 cup pasta water if required. Sprinkle cheese and serve

Nutrients Per Serving: 271 Cal| Total Fat 18.4g| Cholesterol 8.3mg| Sodium 226.9mg| Total Carbohydrate 27.5g| Dietary Fiber 3.6g| Protein 3.9g|Iron 1.4mg| Potassium 268.6mg| Phosphorus 88.5mg

3.3 Linguine with Garlic & Shrimp

Ingredients

- 2 and a half quarts of water

- Peeled and cleaned, Raw shrimp: 3/4 pound

- Linguine: 12 ounces, uncooked

- Olive oil: 2 tablespoons

- Chopped flat-leaf parsley: 1 cup

- Lemon juice: 1 tablespoon

- 2 whole heads of garlic
- Black pepper: 1/4 teaspoon

Instructions

- Cook pasta as per instructions.
- Separate cloves of garlic leave the skin on.
- Heat the garlic cloves in a pan over medium flame, continuously stirring till it becomes soft and darkens. Skin will come off easily. Peel off the skin and set it aside
- Now fry the garlic in olive oil till light golden brown
- Add shrimp, parsley, and cook for two minutes, until shrimp is cooked.
- Add one cup of pasta water and all pasta to the pan. Mix it all up. Add more pasta water if required.
- Add black pepper, lemon juice. Serve.

Nutrients per serving: Calories 322| Protein 20 g| Carbohydrates 47 g| Fat 6 g| Cholesterol 86 mg| Sodium 106 mg| Potassium 298 mg| Phosphorus 220 mg| Calcium 87 mg| Fiber 2.4 g

3.4 Spicy Lemon Pasta

Ingredients

- Lemon zest: 1 teaspoon
- Chopped onion: 1/4 cup
- Butter: 2 teaspoons
- Chopped green bell pepper: 1/4 cup
- Cooked pasta: 3/4 cup
- Fresh lemon juice: 2 tablespoons
- Chopped celery: 1/4 cup
- Onion herb seasoning: 1 teaspoon

Instructions

- In a pan, sauté celery, green bell pepper, and onion in butter.
- Add the sautéed vegetables into hot pasta.
- Add herb seasoning, lemon zest, and lemon juice to the pasta.

Nutrients per serving: Calories 140| Protein 4 g| Carbohydrates 22 g| Fat 4 g| Cholesterol 10 mg| Sodium 44 mg| Potassium 156 mg| Phosphorus 76 mg| Calcium 24 mg| fiber 2.9 g

3.5 Pesto Pronto

Ingredients

- Half cup Mushrooms, thick slices
- White Pasta: 16 oz.
- 1 Yellow Squash, half-moons slices
- Pesto Sauce: 2/3 cup
- 1 Red Bell Pepper, chopped
- 2 Zucchini, half-moons slices
- Olive Oil: 2 tbsp.
- 2 cloves of minced Garlic

Instructions

- Let the oven preheat to 425. Add bell pepper, zucchini, mushrooms, squash, and onion, and a baking sheet. Pour olive oil, coat in an olive oil well. Roast until vegetables are tender. Cook pasta as per instruction.

- In a bowl, add cooked pasta and pesto and roasted vegetable. Coat evenly

- Serve warm.

Nutrition Per Serving: Cal 492| total Fat 18.8g| Cholesterol 5.6mg| Sodium 336.3mg| Total Carbohydrate 66.9g| Dietary Fiber 4.3g| Protein 13.4g| Iron 3.3mg| Potassium 476mg| Phosphorus 237mg

3.6 Pasta with Cheesy Meat Sauce

Ingredients

- Half cup onions, chopped
- Half box pasta, large-shaped
- 4 cups ground beef
- Beef stock: 1 and a half cups, no sodium
- Worcestershire sauce: 2 tablespoons, reduced-sodium
- Beef bouillon: 1 tablespoon, no salt added
- Onion flakes: 1 tablespoon
- Tomato sauce: 1 tablespoon, no salt added
- Pepper jack cheese: ¾ cup shredded

- Half tsp. of Italian seasoning
- Half tsp. of ground black pepper
- One cup of cream cheese softened

Instructions

- Cook pasta as per instructions

- In a pan, cook onions, onion flakes, and ground beef until meat is browned. Drain.

- Add tomato sauce, stock, and bouillon.

- Let it simmer. Add in cooked pasta.

- Turn off the heat, add cheese, cream cheese, and seasonings. Mix pasta until cheese melts.

Nutrition Per Serving: Calories 502 | total Fat 30 g| Saturated Fat 14 g| Trans Fat 1 g| cholesterol 99 mg| Sodium 401 mg| carbohydrates 35 g| Protein 23 g| Phosphorus 278 mg| Potassium 549 mg| Dietary Fiber 1.7 g| Calcium 107 mg

3.7 Spaghetti & Broccoli Carbonara

Ingredients

- Canola oil: 2 teaspoons
- Onions: 1 cup, diced
- One egg whisked
- Non-dairy creamer: 1 cup
- Chicken stock, low-sodium: ¼ cup

- Cooked pasta: 3 cups (spiral noodle)
- 2 cups broccoli, chopped
- Black pepper: 1 teaspoon
- Scallions: ½ cup, chopped

Instructions

- In a pan, sauté onions in oil over medium heat
- In a bowl, add creamer and egg, whisk together.
- Reduce the heat and add the egg mixture into onions, constantly mix until thickens
- Add the broccoli, stock, black pepper, pasta, keep mixing until all heated through.

Nutrition Per Serving: Calories 304 | Total Fat 19 g| Saturated Fat 10 g| Trans Fat 0.5 g| Cholesterol 78 mg| Sodium 141 mg| Carbohydrates 27 g| Protein 9 g| Phosphorus 143 mg| Potassium 287 mg|Dietary Fiber 5.4 g| Calcium 65 mg

3.8 Mediterranean Pasta Salad

Ingredients

- Chopped walnuts: 1 tablespoon(toasted)
- Plain hummus: 2 tablespoons
- Half of a cup diced red bell pepper
- Water: 1 tablespoon
- One cup lightly packed baby kale

- One can unsalted, light tuna in water(drained)
- Half of a cup cooked farfalle (whole-wheat)
- Crumbled feta cheese: 1 tablespoon
- Extra-virgin olive oil: 2 teaspoons
- Juice from ¼ of a lemon

Instructions

- In a mixing bowl, mix water and hummus and set it aside.
- Take a nonstick medium skillet, add extra virgin olive oil and turn the heat on medium.
- Add the chopped bell pepper let it cook for one minute. Then, add kale. Carefully add in the tuna, do not break large fish pieces. Let it warm through for one minute.
- Then add the pasta. Turn off the heat, and add in hummus sauce. Garnish with walnuts, feta. On top of it, drizzle with lemon juice.

Nutrition per serving: 345 calories| total fat 24.5g |carbohydrates 28.3g |protein 33.4g

3.9 Herb Fish with Penne

Ingredients

- Herb Seasoning: 2 teaspoons
- 4 cups of fish cubes

- Small broccoli florets: 2 cups (fresh or frozen)
- Half-and-half: 1 cup(fat-free)
- One cup of penne pasta
- Half teaspoon of Sea Salt
- ½ cup of cheese cubed

Instructions

- In a large saucepan, add pasta and cook as instructed on the packaging. In the last three minutes, add broccoli and fish. Drain it well.
- In the meantime, add half-and-half to a small saucepan on medium flame and let it simmer.
- Lower the heat after, add seasoning, sea salt, and cream cheese. Mix with a whisker until cheese is melted. The sauce is well combined.
- In a bowl, add pasta, broccoli, and fish
- Pour cheese over, lightly coat.
- Serve right away.

Nutrition per serving: 291 calories| total fat 8g |carbohydrates 36g| protein 24g

3.10 Pasta Salad Mediterranean Style

Ingredients

- One pint of cherry tomatoes
- Chinese eggplants: 2 mediums, chopped into small cubes

- Extra virgin olive oil
- One teaspoon of salt
- Pinch of freshly ground black pepper
- 1/4 teaspoon of ground cumin
- 1/4 teaspoon of red pepper flakes
- 1/4 teaspoon of granulated garlic
- 1 package brown of 16 ounces' rice spaghetti, cooked and cooled

Lemon Dressing

- Finely sliced dill: 1 tablespoon
- Finely sliced mint: 1 tablespoon
- Finely sliced parsley: 1 tablespoon
- Finely sliced cilantro: 1 tablespoon

Instructions

- Let the oven pre-heat to 400F, put parchment paper on a rimmed baking sheet
- Add diced eggplant, three tablespoons of extra virgin olive oil, black pepper, red pepper flakes, salt, cherry tomatoes, granulated garlic, and cumin. Mix it well.
- Put this vegetable mix onto the parchment-lined baking tray.
- Bake for about half an hour, until all vegetables, are soft and lightly golden.

- Take out from the oven, and let it cool slightly.

- In a serving bowl, add the cooked, cooled brown rice pasta, drizzle the lemon dressing and mix keep tasting, add as much as to your liking, start slow, then add eggplant mixture/ cherry tomato mix, herbs, and carefully mix everything.

- Taste it and season with additional pepper and salt if required.

- Serve right away or chill in the refrigerator and serve later.

Lemon Dressing

- Half cup of extra virgin olive oil

- 4-6 cloves of garlic minced or press them

- ¼ of teaspoon granulated sugar

- Zest of one lemon

- 1/4 of teaspoon salt

- Freshly ground black pepper

- 1/4 of a cup lemon juice

- Half teaspoon of Dijon mustard

Instructions

- Add all ingredients in a big jar with a lid, cover the top with lid and mix until emulsified.

- Use right away, or store in the fridge to keep cool.

- This dressing works well with other salads and pasta.

Nutrition per serving: 284 calories| total fat 10g | carbohydrates 23g |protein 14g.

3.11 Renal-Friendly Macaroni Salad

Ingredients

- 2 cloves of pressed garlic

- 4 cups, elbow macaroni, cooked

- 1/4 cup onion, chopped

- 1 sweet bell pepper, chopped

- Half cup celery, sliced

- 1 and 1/2 cups low fat mayonnaise

- Apple cider vinegar: 1 teaspoon

- Dijon mustard: 2 teaspoons

- 1 teaspoon honey

- Half teaspoon of black pepper

Instructions

- In a bowl, add bell pepper, macaroni, onions, and celery, mix.

- In another bowl, add mustard, honey, salt, mayonnaise, vinegar mix it well

- Mix these two bowls' ingredients

- Serve chilled.

Nutrient per serving: Calories: 171 g| Protein: 7 g| Carbohydrates: 20.1 g| Fiber: 2.9 g| Total Fat: 2.1 g| Sodium:

101 mg| Phosphorus: 89 mg| Potassium: 98 mg|

3.12 Pasta & Kidney Bean Soup

Ingredients

- One cup chopped onion
- One cup of chopped red bell pepper
- Butter: 1 tablespoon
- 2 cans of red kidney beans
- 4 cups of low-sodium chicken broth
- Six cloves of minced garlic,
- Dried oregano: Half teaspoon
- Olive oil: 2 tablespoons
- Red pepper flakes: half teaspoon
- 1 cup small pasta
- 2 bay leaves
- Salt and black pepper

Instructions

- In a pan, heat butter and olive oil and sauté garlic, red pepper flakes, onion, and oregano, until onion is tender
- Add bell peppers, broth, bay leaves, and beans. Bring it to a boil, then let it simmer for 20 minutes.
- Add pasta to the soup in the last ten minutes. Add salt and pepper.

- Take out bay leaves, and serve.

Nutrient per serving: Calories: 214 g| Protein: 12 g| Carbohydrates: 22 g| Fiber: 2.2 g| Total Fat: 6.5 g| Sodium: 204 mg| Phosphorus: 132 mg| Potassium: 245 mg|

3.13 Healthy Kidney Bean Pasta

Ingredients

- One Tablespoon of olive oil
- Cooked penne pasta: 2 cups
- Peas: 1 cup
- Chopped one onion
- Kidney beans: 2 cups
- Sea salt
- Three cloves of pressed garlic
- One Tablespoon of white wine vinegar

Instructions

- Cook pasta as per instructions. Set it aside.
- In a pan, sauté olive oil, onion, vinegar, garlic, cook for five minutes
- Add the kidney beans; peas continue to cook for three minutes, stirring continuously.
- Add the pasta and mix well.
- Serve immediately.

Nutrient per serving: Calories: 234 g| Protein: 14 g| Carbohydrates: 18.5 g| Fiber: 1.9 g| Total Fat: 4 g| Sodium:

109 mg| Phosphorus: 98 mg| Potassium: 145 mg|

3.14 Chilled Veggie & Shrimp Noodle Salad

Ingredients

- Mushrooms chopped: 2 cups
- One pound of cooked spaghetti
- Chili oil: 2 teaspoons
- Sliced scallions: 1 cup
- Broccoli florets: 2 cups
- Carrots: 1 cup
- 4 cups of cooked shrimp
- Sesame oil: 2 tablespoons
- Garlic: 2 tablespoons chopped
- Half cup of rice wine vinegar
- Zest of lime: 1 tablespoon
- Ginger: 1 tablespoon, chopped
- Soy sauce, low-sodium: ¼ cup
- ¼ cup fresh lime juice

Instructions

- Mix all ingredients in a bowl.
- Toss everything together and serve

Nutrition Per Serving: Calories 254 | Total Fat 11 g| Saturated Fat 2 g| Trans Fat 0 g| Cholesterol 84 mg| Sodium 433 mg| Carbohydrates 27 g| Protein 13 g| Phosphorus 229 mg| Potassium 325 mg| Dietary Fiber 3 g| Calcium 73 mg

3.15 Macaroni & Cheese

Ingredients

- Unsalted butter: 2 tablespoons
- Rotini pasta: 1 cup uncooked
- Low-fat milk: half cup
- Grated parmesan cheese: 3 tablespoons
- Half cup and a little more of cream cheese, reduced-fat
- Crushed red pepper flakes: 1/8 teaspoon
- Black pepper: 1/4 teaspoon
- One clove of pressed garlic

Instructions

- Cook pasta as per instructions, without salt.
- In a pan, sauté garlic for one minute in butter. Add cream cheese, milk, whisk well.
- Simmer the sauce on low heat.
- Add black pepper, red pepper flakes to taste.
- Add cooked pasta to the sauce.

Nutrients per serving: Calories 266| Protein 9 g| Carbohydrates 26 g| Fat 14 g| Cholesterol 43 mg| Sodium 237 mg| Potassium 222 mg| Phosphorus 188 mg| Calcium 147 mg| Fiber 2.3 g

3.16 Easy Pantry Pasta

Ingredients

- Canned cannellini beans: 1 cup

- One and a half cup of dried pasta

- Half cup of tuna packed in water, low-sodium

- Tomato sauce: half cup (no salt added)

- Chicken broth: half cup, low-sodium

- Olive oil: 2 tablespoons

- Roasted red peppers jarred: 1/3 cup

- Onion powder: half teaspoon

- Garlic powder: half teaspoon

- Dried basil: half teaspoon

- Green peas: half cup

- Parmesan cheese: 1 tablespoon

- Dried oregano: 1/4 teaspoon

Instructions

- Cook pasta as per instructions, without salt. Reserve half a cup of pasta water.

- Slice the red peppers.

- In a pan, add remaining ingredients, do not add cheese and peas.

- Add pasta to the sauce and mix well. Add pasta water to the sauce. If the sauce is too thick

- Add parmesan cheese and green peas mix well. Enjoy

Nutrients per serving: Calories 344| Protein 18 g| Carbohydrates 50 g| Fat 8 g| Cholesterol 13 mg| Sodium 290 mg| Potassium 542 mg| Phosphorus 230 mg| Calcium 76 mg| Fiber 5.4 g

3.17 Pasta with Cauliflower

Ingredients

- One and a half cups of chicken broth, low-sodium

- Olive oil: 2 tablespoons

- One onion, chopped

- One cauliflower, medium head, chopped

- 3 cloves of garlic, minced

- Black pepper: 1/4 teaspoon

- 2 cups of linguine, uncooked

- Fresh parsley: 2 tablespoons

- Crushed red pepper: 1/4 teaspoon

Instructions

- In a pan, sauté garlic and onion in oil until translucent

- Add red pepper, cauliflower, and black pepper and sauté for five minutes.

- Add broth and let it boil. Lower the heat to simmer till cauliflower is tender.

- Cook pasta as per instructions, without salt

- Put the drained pasta back in the pot add cauliflower broth to the pasta so it will not stick

- Add pasta in a serving bowl, add cauliflower broth and serve.

Nutrients per serving: Calories 298| Protein 12 g| Carbohydrates 49 g| Fat 6 g| Cholesterol 4 mg| Sodium 133 mg| Potassium 420 mg| phosphorus 231 mg| calcium 89 mg| Fiber 8.6 g

3.18 Creamy Orzo & Vegetables

Ingredients

- Olive oil: 2 tablespoons
- Frozen green peas: half cup
- One clove of minced garlic
- One zucchini, chopped
- One carrot, shredded
- Curry powder: 1 teaspoon
- Chicken broth, low-sodium: 3 cups
- One diced small onion
- Black pepper: 1/4 teaspoon
- Salt: 1/4 teaspoon
- Fresh parsley: 2 tablespoons
- Orzo pasta: 1 cup, uncooked
- Grated Parmesan cheese: 1/4 cup

Instructions

- In a pan, sauté onion, carrots, garlic, and zucchini for five minutes.
- Add broth, curry powder, and salt. Let it boil.
- Add pasta and bring to a boil. Cover it and let it simmer. Cook, often stirring for ten minutes, till pasta is cooked.
- Add chopped parsley, cheese, and frozen peas.
- Heat until all vegetables are heated through. Add more broth if required. Add black pepper and serve.

Nutrients per serving: Calories 176| Protein 10 g| carbohydrates 25 g| Fat 4 g| Cholesterol 4 mg| Sodium 193 mg| Potassium 170 mg| Phosphorus 68 mg| Calcium 53 mg| Fiber 2.6 g

3.19 Lemon Orzo Spring Salad

Ingredients

- Olive oil: ¼ cup+ 2 tbsp.
- Orzo pasta: ¾ cup
- Green peppers: ¼ cup, chopped
- Parmesan cheese: 3 tablespoons
- Yellow peppers: ¼ cup, chopped
- Half cup onion, chopped
- Fresh lemon juice: 3 tablespoons
- Lemon zest: 1 teaspoon
- Zucchini: 2 cups, cubed
- Red peppers: ¼ cup, chopped
- Rosemary: 2 tablespoons, chopped
- Black pepper: half teaspoon
- Red pepper flakes: half teaspoon

- Dried oregano: Half teaspoon

Instructions

- Cook pasta as per instructions, without salt
- In a pan, sauté zucchini, onions, peppers, until translucent, with two tbsp. of oil
- In a bowl, mix lemon zest, juice, red pepper flakes, rosemary, oregano, ¼ cup olive oil, pepper, and cheese.
- Add pasta and vegetables and coat well
- Serve at room temperature.

Nutrition Per Serving: Calories 330 | Total Fat 22 g| saturated Fat 4 g| trans Fat 0 g| Cholesterol 3 mg| sodium 79 mg| Carbohydrates 28 g| Protein 6 g| Phosphorus 134 mg| Potassium 376 mg| Dietary Fiber 5 g| Calcium 67 mg

3.20 Garlicky Penne Pasta with Green Beans

Ingredients

- 2 tablespoons olive oil
- Butter: 2 tablespoon
- Red pepper flakes: 1/8 teaspoon
- Tabasco hot sauce: 1/4 teaspoon
- Shredded parmesan cheese: 1/4 cup
- 4 cups green beans
- Six garlic cloves, minced
- Black pepper: half teaspoon

- Lemon juice: 2 teaspoons
- One cup of uncooked penne pasta

Instructions

- Cook pasta as per instructions, without salt
- In a pan, sauté red pepper flakes, garlic in butter and olive oil for 2 to 3 minutes.
- Add green beans, lemon juice, black pepper, tabasco sauce, and cook for six minutes until tender crispy.
- Add pasta. And toss.

Nutrients per serving: Calories 258| Protein 9 g| Carbohydrates 33 g| Fat 10 g| Cholesterol 13 mg| Sodium 93 mg| Potassium 258 mg| Phosphorus 168 mg| Calcium 83 mg| Fiber 4.8 g

3.21 Italian Style Vegetables & Pasta with Chicken

Ingredients

- One cup of cooked pasta twists
- Olive oil: 1 tablespoon
- Chopped onion: 1/4 cup
- Half teaspoon of garlic powder
- Half cup of chopped green bell pepper
- Half cup broccoli florets
- ¼ cup of chicken, cooked, diced
- Fresh basil: 1 tablespoon
- Dried rosemary: 1 teaspoon

- Red pepper flakes: 1/4 teaspoon

- Cornstarch: 2 teaspoons

- Salt: 1/8 teaspoon

- Chicken broth, low-sodium: 1/4 cup

Instructions

- In a pan, fry onion, broccoli, bell pepper. Add basil, garlic powder, rosemary, salt, red pepper flakes.

- Add in the cooked chicken.

- Mix cornstarch with chicken broth, and add to chicken and vegetable mix. Cook till slightly thickened. Add in the hot cooked pasta.

- Serve.

Nutrients per serving: Calories 250| Protein 15 g| Carbohydrates 28 g| Fat 9 g| Cholesterol 22 mg| Sodium 265 mg| Potassium 329 mg| Phosphorus 140 mg| Calcium 72 mg| Fiber 3.7 g

3.22 Green Pesto Pasta

Ingredients

- Fresh basil leaves: 2 cups

- Half cup and a little more of uncooked spaghetti

- 4 cloves of garlic

- Extra virgin olive oil: 1/4 cup

- Black pepper: 1/4 teaspoon

- Grated Parmesan cheese: 2 tablespoons

Instructions

- Cook pasta as per instructions, without salt. Drain.

- In a food processor, add Parmesan cheese, basil leaves, and garlic, chop them. Slowly add olive oil and pulse.

- Add black pepper. Add basil sauce to pasta and coat evenly.

Nutrients per serving: Calories 303| Protein 8 g| Carbohydrates 34 g| Fat 15 g| Cholesterol 2 mg| sodium 47 mg| Potassium 170 mg| Phosphorus 145 mg| Calcium 92 mg| Fiber 5.5 g

3.23 Classic Beef Stroganoff with Egg Noodles

Ingredients

- One egg whisked

- Onions: 1 cup, finely chopped

- Low-fat mayonnaise: 1 tablespoon

- Worcestershire sauce: 2 tablespoons, reduced-sodium

- Tomato sauce: 1 tablespoon, no salt added

- 4 cups of ground beef

- Breadcrumbs: ¼ cup

- Bouillon beef: 4 teaspoons, reduced-sodium

- Olive oil: 3 tablespoons

- Sour cream: ¼ cup

- Flour: 2 tablespoons

- Rosemary: 1 tablespoon, chopped
- Water: 3 cups
- Wide egg noodles, cooked
- Ground black pepper: 1 teaspoon
- Cubed butter: 2 tablespoons unsalted, cold
- 2 tablespoons chives
- Parsley: ¼ cup

Instructions

- In a bowl, add beef, egg, and spices, half of the black pepper mix well and make small meatballs.
- In a pan, brown the meatballs.
- In another pan, add flour, oil, and mix, add black pepper, bouillon, water, mix till thickened.
- Mix this sauce with chives, sour cream, and meatballs. Serve with egg noodles/.

Nutrition Per Serving: Calories 490 | total Fat 32 g| saturated Fat 11 g| trans Fat 1 g| Cholesterol 120 mg| sodium 598 mg| Carbohydrates 30 g| Protein 20 g| Phosphorus 230 mg| Potassium 423 mg| Dietary Fiber 1.8 g| Calcium 56 mg

3.24 Easy Chicken & Pasta Dinner

Ingredients

- Half cup of chicken breast, cooked, cut into strips
- Olive oil: 1 tablespoon
- One cup sliced zucchini
- Half cup of sliced red bell pepper
- Italian dressing, low-sodium: 3 tablespoons
- Cooked pasta: 2 cups

Instructions

- In a skillet, sauté peppers, zucchini in olive oil until tender. Set it aside
- In another pan, heat the chicken and pasta. Add Italian dressing and vegetables, mix well and serve.

Nutrients per serving: Calories 400| Protein 30 g| Carbohydrates 45 g| Fat 11 g| Cholesterol 60 mg| Sodium 328 mg| Potassium 455 mg| Phosphorus 270 mg| Calcium 33 mg| Fiber 3.5 g

3.25 Alfredo Sauce Pasta

Ingredients

- Unsalted butter: 1/4 cup
- Half cup of cream cheese, cut into cubes
- Soy milk: 3/4 cup
- White pepper: 1/4 teaspoon
- Garlic powder: 1/8 teaspoon
- Half cup grated Cheese

Instructions

- In a pan, mix all the ingredients on low heat until well combined.

- Add in the cooked pasta and coat well.

- Enjoy.

Nutrients per serving: Calories 124| Protein 3 g| Carbohydrates 3 g| Fat 12 g| Cholesterol 36 mg| Sodium 153 mg| Potassium 65 mg| Phosphorus 70 mg| Calcium 87 mg| Fiber 0 g

3.26 Roasted Vegetable & Chicken Pasta

Ingredients

Vegetables

- One pint sliced mushrooms

- One chopped zucchini

- Half sliced onion

- One cup cherry tomatoes

- 1 chopped yellow squash

- One small broccoli, chop into small pieces

- Olive oil: ¼ cup

- Garlic powder: ¼ teaspoon

- One red pepper, diced

- Onion powder: ¼ teaspoon

- Coarse kosher salt: 1 teaspoon

- Half teaspoon of pepper

Pasta

- Extra virgin olive oil: ¼ cup

- Salt and pepper to taste

- 1 box of pasta, cooked

- Cheese: ⅔ cup shredded

Chicken

- Extra virgin olive oil: 1 tablespoon

- 6 cups of chicken breasts

- Half teaspoon of pepper

- One full hand kale

- Half teaspoon of coarse kosher salt

Instructions

Vegetables

- Let the oven preheat to 350.

- On a baking sheet, place mushrooms, zucchini, broccoli, squash, red pepper, onion, and tomatoes. Sprinkle onion powder, pepper, garlic powder, olive oil, and salt. Mix well

- Roast for half an hour, stirring every ten minutes.

Chicken

- Cut the chicken into cubes

- In a pan, sauté chicken with pepper and salt in olive oil

- Cook chicken for six minutes or till its cooked.

- Add kale to the chicken pan and cook for 20 seconds till kale has wilted.

Pasta

- Add salt, pepper, cheese to hot pasta and mix well

Assemble

- In a big bowl, add chicken, roasted vegetables, and pasta

- Taste and adjust seasoning.

- Serve right away

Nutrient per serving: Calories 282 g| Protein: 15 g| Carbohydrates: 21.4 g| Fiber: 2.7 g| Total Fat: 5 g| Sodium: 209 mg| Phosphorus: 145 mg| Potassium: 189 mg|

3.27 Roasted Red Pepper Pesto

Ingredients

- 2 cloves of garlic, cut in half

- 1 tsp. balsamic vinegar

- One jar of red bell peppers, roasted, drained

- Fresh basil: ¼ cup

- Pepper to taste

- Olive oil: ¼ cup

- One packet of Ravioli, low sodium

Instructions

- In a food processor, add all ingredients, except pasta. Pulse on high for 30 seconds, till smooth. Adjust seasoning

- Cook ravioli as per instruction.

- Coat the cooked ravioli with sauce and enjoy.

Nutrition per serving: Calories 526 kcals| Sodium 487 mg| Protein 17 g| Potassium 294 mg| Fat 37 g| calcium 66 mg |Carbohydrates 31 g| Phosphorus 186 mg| Fiber 2 g| Cholesterol 130mg

3.28 Chicken and Bow-Tie Pasta

Ingredients

- Cayenne pepper: 1/4 teaspoon

- Cooked bow-tie pasta: 3 cups

- Chicken broth, low sodium: 1 cup

- 2 cloves of minced garlic

- Olive oil: 1/4 cup

- Chopped red pepper: 1 cup

- One and a half cups chopped broccoli

- One cup of chicken breast, cut into strips

- Half cup of chopped green onions

- White wine: 3/4 cup

- Ground basil: 1 teaspoon

Instructions

- In a skillet, sauté garlic.

- Add chicken and brown it.

- Add all the remaining ingredients and let it simmer for 15 minutes

- Mix with cooked pasta.

Nutrition per serving: Calories 258 kcals| Sodium 50 mg| protein 13 g| Potassium 338 mg| Fat 10 g| Calcium 43 mg| Carbohydrates 25 g| phosphorus 173 mg| Fiber 5 g| cholesterol 22 mg|

3.29 Chicken Fusilli Salad

Dressing

- White pepper: half teaspoon
- Half cup of olive oil
- Vinegar: 1/4 cup
- Honey: 1 teaspoon
- Basil: 1/4 teaspoon

Salad

- Half cup of chopped red pepper
- Fusilli pasta cooked: 3 cups
- Shredded lettuce: 2 cups
- Half cup of cooked peas
- 1 carrot, thin slices
- Sliced zucchini: 1 cup
- One cup of diced cooked chicken

Instructions

- In a jar, add ingredients of dressing, shake and mix well, chill in the fridge for two hours.
- In a bowl, add zucchini, pasta, carrot, chicken, red pepper, and peas, mix well
- Add dressing, and mix well

Nutrient per serving: Calories 477 kcals| Sodium 65 mg| Protein 18 g| Potassium 446 mg| Fat 29 g| Calcium 31 mg| Carbohydrates 39 g| Phosphorus 239 mg| Fiber 8 g| Cholesterol 33 mg

3.30 Pad Thai

Ingredients

- Vegetable oil: 3 tablespoons
- Honey: 2 tablespoons
- 2 cloves of minced garlic
- Chinese chives: 6 tbsp.
- Half cups of extra-firm tofu
- Carrot & cabbage slaw mix: 1 cup
- One lime
- 4 tbsp. Of unseasoned rice vinegar
- Reduced-sodium soy sauce: 1 tablespoon
- Dried noodles, rice stick: 7 ounces
- Red chili sauce: 1 tablespoon
- One and a half cups of bean sprouts
- 2 eggs

Instructions

- Chop all the vegetables and tofu.
- In a boiled pot of water, turn off the heat, add rice noodles, separate them, soak for five minutes, drain and set it aside.

- In a small bowl, mix honey, chili sauce, vinegar, soy sauce. Set it aside

- In a wok, sauté tofu until it begins to brown for two minutes. Set it aside

- Add one tbsp. of oil and garlic in the wok fry a few seconds, add the noodles and chives, fry for few seconds. Add in the honey mix, add slaw mix, bean sprouts. Cook for two minutes.

- Cook eggs and coat with noodles, add tofu, and mix.

- Serve immediately.

Nutrients per serving: Calories 436| Protein 9 g| Carbohydrates 64 g| Fat 16 g| Cholesterol 93 mg| Sodium 430 mg| Potassium 445 mg| Phosphorus 163 mg| Calcium 81 mg| Fiber 2.8 g

3.31 Spaghetti Squash Parmigiano

Ingredients

- 2 cloves of minced garlic

- One small spaghetti squash

- 1 onion

- Red chili flakes: 1/8 teaspoon

- Olive oil: 4 tablespoons

- Parmigiano-Reggiano cheese, grated: 3/4 cup

- Black pepper: 1/4 teaspoon

Instructions

- Let the oven preheat to 375° F.

- Stab squash with a fork—microwave for five minutes. Cut in half and remove seeds.

- Pour olive oil over the squash, and bake for 50 minutes.

- Take out squash. Let it cool down.

- In a skillet, sauté onion and garlic for 2 to 3 minutes. Turn off the heat.

- With a fork, pulp the squash and add to skillet. Add cheese, red flakes, and black pepper. Mix to combine

Nutrients per serving: Calories 138| Protein 5 g| Carbohydrates 7 g| Fat 10 g| Cholesterol 11 mg| Sodium 200 mg| Potassium 160 mg| Phosphorus 110 mg| Calcium 162 mg|Fiber 1.7 g

3.32 Pancit

Ingredients

- Carrots: 2 cups, shredded

- 3 cloves of minced garlic

- Half cup of onion, minced

- 4 cups of shredded cabbage

- 2 chopped green onions

- olive oil: 1 tablespoon

- 3 stalks of celery

- 1 cup cooked chicken

- 2 cups of frozen snow peas

- Chicken broth, low-sodium: 4 cups

- Rice sticks(noodles) of 16 ounces
- Half teaspoon of black pepper
- Soy sauce, reduced-sodium: 1 tablespoon

Instructions

- In a skillet, sauté onion, garlic in olive oil until tender
- Add in the chicken and soy sauce. Add three cups of broth and let it boil
- Add noodles, cook for 15 minutes, until translucent but do not overcook
- Add the vegetables, cook until cabbage becomes tender.
- Serve right away and add lemon juice.

Nutrients per serving: Calories 255| Protein 12 g| Carbohydrates 41 g| Fat 5 g| cholesterol 59 mg| Sodium 220 mg| Potassium 373 mg| Phosphorus 141 mg| calcium 49 mg| Fiber 2.7 g

3.33 Garlic Shrimp Zoodles

Ingredients

- Medium shrimp 3/4 pounds, deveined
- Olive oil: 1 tablespoon
- Garlic minced: 3-4 cloves
- Two medium zucchini
- Red chili flakes
- Chopped parsley

- Salt & pepper, to taste
- One lemon: Juice and zest

Instruction

- First off, spiralizer the zucchini and set it aside
- Add lemon juice, the olive oil, zest of lemon to a skillet on medium flame. Then add the shrimp until the pan is hot. Cook 1 minute per side of the shrimp.
- Add red chili flakes, garlic. Cook for a full minute, always stirring.
- Add the zoodles and toss for 2-3 minutes until cooked and warmed thoroughly
- Sprinkle with the sliced parsley and season with pepper and salt. Serve hot.

Nutrition per serving: Kcal 276| Fat 10g|Carbohydrates 9g|Protein 12g

3.34 Zucchini Noodles with Roasted Halibut

Ingredients

- Wild halibut of 6 ounces
- Olive Oil
- Red curry paste: 1 tablespoon
- One package of zucchini noodles
- Salt, pepper to taste
- Two minced cloves of garlic
- Four sliced scallions, sliced

- Half of cup of cilantro
- Two inches of ginger root(grated)
- Red pepper flakes: 1/4 teaspoon

Instructions

- Put a skillet over medium flame and heat the coconut oil.
- Add the zoodles, curry paste, ginger and, garlic. Cook for about four minutes until the noodles are tender, keep stirring— season taste.
- Put another skillet over medium flame and heat the coconut oil. Place skin-side down the fish. Season with red pepper flakes and salt.
- Turn on the broiler.
- Cook for seven minutes, then move to the broiler. Broil for five minutes or until the fish is completely cooked
- Add the noodles with scallions and cilantro and stir to combine.
- Place on a plate, top with fish, and serve.

Nutrition per serving :196 calories| total fat 1.1g |carbohydrates 24.6g |protein 23.5g

3.35 Red Bell Pepper Basil Garlic Chicken

Ingredients

- One pound of skinless chicken breasts
- Olive oil: 2 tablespoons
- Half onion, diced
- Three minced garlic cloves
- Red bell peppers: one and a half cups
- Basil: 1 cup
- Red chili flakes: 1/4 teaspoon
- Four zucchini and courgette: spiralizer into noodles
- Salt & pepper, to taste

Instructions

- Pound, the chicken breast to achieve the same overall thickness. When finished, sprinkle a touch of salt and pepper on either side.
- In a wide skillet, add one tablespoon of olive oil, warm it. stir in the chicken and fry each side for a few minutes until golden brown
- When the chicken has been cooked completely and browned, remove it from the skillet and put aside for the time being, on a separate dish.
- Using the same skillet, add olive oil and sauté the onion until it becomes translucent for around five minutes. Then add the garlic and Sautee for about another minute.
- Add the basil and tomatoes in the pan and add salt, pepper, and

then red pepper flakes to season.

- Simmer for ten minutes until the sauce thickens. Please make sure you mix regularly.

- Send the chicken back to the skillet together with the zoodles for a couple of minutes so they can soak up the sauce. Serve hot

Nutrition per serving: Kcal 251| Fat: 8 g| Carbs 12g |Protein: 27g

3.36 Mac Stuffed Sweet Potatoes

Ingredients

- One sweet potato (leached)

- ¼ cup whole-grain penne pasta

- 1 tsp tomato paste, no salt added

- Olive oil 1 tsp

- ¼ teaspoon minced garlic

- 1 tbsp. soy milk

Instructions

- Cut the sweet potato in two and holes it 3-4 times with fork.

- Spray the sweet potato halves with olive oil and cook in the Preheated to 375 F oven for about 25-30 minutes or when the vegetables are tender.

- In the meantime, cook penne pasta, tomato paste, minced garlic, and soy milk.

- When the sweet potatoes are baked, spoon out the vegetable

meat and spice it up with a penne pasta combination.

- Cover the sweet potatoes with the pasta mix.

Nutrition per serving: 105 calories| 2.7g protein|17.8g carbohydrates|2.8g fat|3g fiber|0mg cholesterol

3.37 Pasta Soup

Ingredients

- 2 oz. whole-grain pasta

- ½ cup corn kernels

- 1 oz. carrot, shredded

- 3 oz. celery stalk, chopped

- 2 cups low-sodium chicken stock

- 1 teaspoon ground black pepper

Instructions

- Bring the chicken stock to boil and add shredded carrot and celery stalk. Simmer the liquid for 5 minutes.

- After this, add corn kernels, ground black pepper, and pasta. Stir the soup well.

- Simmer it on the medium heat for 8 minutes.

Nutrition per serving: 263 calories|11.8g protein|29.6g carbohydrates| 2.6g fat|9.4g fiber|0mg cholesterol| 200mg sodium|273mg potassium.

3.38 Lunch Tuna Salad

Ingredients

- Five ounces of dried, soaked tuna in water
- 1 spoon of red vinegar
- Olive oil for 1 tbsp.
- 1/4 cup green, minced onions
- Arugula two cups
- 1 tbsp. low-fat, grated parmesan
- A squeeze of black pepper
- Half cup of pasta, cooked

Instructions

- Mix the tuna and the vinegar, oil, arugula, pasta, green onions, and black pepper in a bowl. Mix.
- Split into Three pans, spray on top with parmesan and serve for lunch.

Nutrition per serving: calories 200| fat 4 g| fiber 4mg| carbs 14 g| protein 7g | potassium 217 mg| phosphorous 113 mg

3.39 Veggie Soup

Ingredients

- Two olive oil teaspoons
- 1 and 1/2 carrot cups, shredded
- Six cloves of garlic, minced
- 1 cup of yellow, chopped onion
- 1 cup of diced celery
- Low-sodium chicken stock: 4 cups
- Four Cups of Water

- 1 and 1/2 cups pasta
- two tablespoons of parsley
- 1/4 cup low-fat, grated parmesan

Instructions

- Over medium-high warm, warm a pan with the oil, add garlic, mix and simmer for 1 minute.
- Add the onion, celery, and carrot, stir, and roast for 7 minutes.
- Add onion, water and pasta, stir, bring to a boil and simmer for Eight more minutes over moderate flame.
- Split into cups, top, and serve each with parsley and parmesan.

Nutrition per serving: calories 212| fat 4 g| fiber 4 g| carbs 13 g| protein 8 g| potassium 198 mg| phosphorous 109 mg

3.40 Italian Pasta

Ingredients

- One pound penne pasta, cooked
- Three cloves of garlic, diced
- Olive oil, Two tablespoons
- Three carrots, cut
- One bell pepper red, diced
- 1 bell pepper purple, chopped
- One cup of cherry tomatoes halved
- black pepper
- 2/3 cup soy milk

- Two teaspoons low-fat, grated parmesan

Instructions

- Over medium-high heat, warm a skillet with the oil, add the garlic, stir and simmer for 2 minutes.

- Add the vegetables, stir and simmer for an additional four minutes.

- Add the bell peppers, yellow and red, and combine and roast for 5 minutes.

- Add black pepper, cherry tomatoes, milk, parmesan, pasta, mix, and serve

Nutrition per serving: calories 221|fat 7.8 g| fiber 2.2mg|carbs 15 g| protein 12 potassium 121 mg| phosphorous 108 mg

3.41 Creamy Garlic Pasta with Roasted Tomatoes

Ingredients

- 3 cups cherry tomatoes (halved)

- One and ¼ cup of pasta

- Olive oil

- Two medium shallots

- 8 large cloves minced garlic

- Sea salt and black pepper

- 3-4 Tbsp. all-purpose flour

- 2-1/2 cups of broth

Instructions

- Preheat oven to 400 degrees F (204 C) and toss tomatoes in a bit of olive oil and sea salt. Place cut side up on a parchment-lined baking sheet and bake for 20 minutes while preparing the rest of the dish. Then set aside.

- Bring a large pot of water to a boil and cook pasta according to package Instructions, and set aside.

- In the meantime, prepare the sauce. In a large skillet over medium-low heat, add 1 Tbsps. Olive oil and the garlic and shallot. Add a pinch of salt and black pepper and frequently stir, cooking for 3-4 minutes until softened and fragrant.

- Stir in flour and mix with a whisk. Once combined, slowly whisk in the almond milk a little at a time, so clumps don't form. Add another healthy pinch of salt and black pepper, bring to a simmer and continue cooking for another 4-5 minutes to thicken. Taste and adjust seasonings as needed,

- If you want an ultra-creamy sauce, transfer the sauce to a blender to blend it until creamy and smooth. Place back in the pan and reduce heat to a low simmer until the desired thickness is achieved.

- Once the sauce is to your desired thickness, taste and adjusts seasonings as needed, then add pasta and roasted tomatoes and stir.

- Serve immediately and garnish with extra black pepper, fresh basil, or vegan parmesan cheese. Best when fresh, but will keep for up to 2 days in the fridge.

Nutrition per serving: Calories: 379| carbohydrates: 64 g| Protein: 11.5 g| Fat: 9 g| saturated Fat: 0.8 g| trans Fat: 0 g| sodium: 360 mg| fiber: 8.5 g

3.42 Ratatouille-Stuffed Shells

Ingredients

- 2 cups of uncooked jumbo pasta shells

- One tablespoon olive oil

- 3/4 cup chopped onion

- One tablespoon minced garlic

- 1 and a half cups diced eggplant

- 1 cup diced red bell pepper

- 3/4 cup diced zucchini

- 3/4 cup chopped plum tomato

- 1 3/4 cups, Low-Sodium marinara sauce

- Half cup plus 2 Tbsp. torn fresh basil, divided

- 3/4 teaspoon freshly ground black pepper

- Half teaspoon kosher salt

- One cup shredded vegan cheese

Instructions

- Preheat 450 ° F oven.

- Cook spaghetti, omitting salt and fat in compliance with product instructions.

- Heat oil medium-high in a large skillet. Add onion and garlic. Cook for 4 minutes, stirring regularly. Add aubergine and pepper.

- Cover and prepare the courgettes, tomatoes, cook for 4 min. Stir in 1 cup of marinara, half cup of basil, black pepper, and salt and remove the pan from the sun.

- Spray oil on ceramic baker. Place marinara over the bottom of the dish remaining 3/4 cup. Spoon into pasta around two tablespoons of the vegetable blend. Sprinkle with cheese; place the shells complete in the dish—Bake 12 minutes at 450 ° F. Top with basil.

Nutrition per serving: Calories 370 | fat 11.8g | sat fat 4.1g | Mono fat 4.3g|Poly fat 1.4g | Protein 16g | Carbohydrate 30g|Fiber 6g | Cholesterol 20mg | iron 4mg |Sodium 486mg | calcium 275mg | Sugars 11g |

3.43 Capers Pasta Salad

Ingredients

- 2 cups rotini pasta

- ⅓ cup extra-virgin olive oil

- 2 pints' cherry or grape tomatoes

- ½ teaspoon fine sea salt

- One cup of mozzarella "pearls,"

- Several sprigs of fresh basil

Instructions

- Bring a big pot of water to a boil and prepare the pasta until ready for use. Set it aside.

- When the pasta has cooked, mix oil, tomatoes, salt on medium-high heat, in a Dutch oven. Cover the pot. Cook till the most tomatoes has soften, and also the olive oil has a faint red shade (around 6 to 12 minutes).

- Take off the heat and add in the pasta you have prepared. let the mixture to cool when chopping basil for a few minutes. We do not want to melt the cheese when in touch so wait until the next phase is mild (not hot) for your pasta.

- Drop from the pasta the mozzarella balls as well as basil. Taste the vinegar and apply extra vinegar or salt if it is not amazing yet. Let the combination sit for about 20 minutes of better taste so that the pasta will handle more sauce.

Nutrition per serving: Calories 552|Total Fat 33.9g | saturated Fat 11.5g| Monounsaturated Fat 16.7g |Cholesterol 50.6mg |Sodium 681.8mg |Total Carbohydrate 47.1g |Dietary Fiber 8.4g |Sugars 8.3g | protein 20g

3.44 Lemony Collard Greens Pasta

Ingredients

- One cup of fresh collard greens

- ⅓ or more of a package of whole wheat thin spaghetti or "spaghetti."

- Three tablespoons pine nuts

- Olive oil

- Two small cloves garlic, pressed

- Big pinch red pepper flakes

- Sea salt and black pepper

- 2 tbsp. of Parmesan cheese

- ½ or more of a lemon, cut into wedges

Instructions

- Carry a large pot of salted water and cook the pasta as instructed.

- Take the middle rib out of a green leaves. Place some greens together and roll them into the form of a cigar. As small as practicable (1/8″ to 1/4″), break through the pin. Give them a good chopping, so the branches aren't too fat. Shake the greens up.

- Heat a heavy-bottom pot over moderate flame and roast the pine nuts till they are golden and scented.

- Switch to medium heat and mix in an olive oil tablespoon. Sprinkle the garlic and whisk in red pepper. When the oil is dark enough to shine, pour it onto the greens. Add salt to the greens. Mix regularly, sauté the greens for around three minutes, and not to make them clump.

- Let the fire of the pan. Shift the vegetables into the pasta pot and add pasta water if necessary, with a second drizzle of olive oil.

- Separate into plates and put two larger citrus wedges, an individual on top of pine nuts and paramedic shavings.

Nutrition per serving: Calories 584| Total Fat 29.2g |Saturated Fat 6.1g |Trans Fat 0g |polyunsaturated Fat 8.5g | cholesterol 9.7mg |Sodium 238.1mg | Total Carbohydrate 68.1g |Dietary Fiber 14.3g | Sugars 2.8g |Protein 22.1g

4.45 Easy One-Pot Pasta

Ingredients

- One cup dry pasta
- 2 garlic cloves, minced
- Half yellow onion, thinly sliced
- 1 small zucchini, chopped and quartered
- 1/4 cup of mushrooms, sliced
- Half teaspoon red pepper flakes
- Half teaspoon kosher salt

- 1 and 1/4 cup pasta sauce of choice, no salt added
- 2 half cups of water
- ¼ cup kale

Instructions

- In a large pot (or pan with deep surfaces), incorporate the uncooked pasta. In addition to the kale, combine the remaining ingredients well. Blend well. Take the pot to a high heat boil.

- Reduce heat to a medium-low until cooked and cook pasta until al-dente for 10-14 minutes. Add the blend to the bottom of the pan after 2 minutes to avoid sticking.

- Turn off the heat and bring it into the pasta, the kale. When the kale has cooled, add the pasta into cups.

Nutrition per serving: Calories 378|Fat 5g |Sodium 272mg|Potassium 245 mg| Carbohydrates 72g|Fiber 11g|Sugar 6.7 g| Protein 15g| Calcium 164mg|Iron 4.9mg

3.46 Scampi Linguine

Ingredients

- 1 clove of garlic, minced
- One tbsp. of olive oil
- Dry white wine: ¼ cup
- 1 tbsp. of lemon juice
- 1 tsp of basil

- Half cup of dry linguine
- 2 cups of shrimp, peeled, cleaned
- Chopped fresh parsley: 1 tbsp.

Instructions

- In a skillet, cook shrimp and garlic until shrimp turns pink
- Add basil, wine, parsley, and lemon juice. Cook for five minutes
- Cook pasta as per instructions, without salt
- Coat pasta with shrimp and serve

Nutrition per serving: Calories 208 kcal |Sodium 86 mg| Protein 15 g| Potassium 189 mg| Phosphorus 167 mg| Calcium 140 mg | Fat 5 g| Water 40 g| Carbohydrates 26 g

3.47 15-Minute Sesame Ginger Noodles

Ingredients

- One sliced green onion
- Baby bock choy: 3 cups, quarters
- Half pack rice noodles

Sauce

- 3 tbsp. low sodium soy sauce
- 2 cloves of garlic, chopped
- Maple syrup: 2 tbsp.
- Sesame oil: 2 tsp

- Crushed red chili: 2 tsp
- 2 tbsp. of ginger, chopped

Instructions

- In a bowl, mix all the ingredients of the sauce, set aside
- Boil rice noodles as per package instructions set it aside.
- In a pan, add sauce and cook for two minutes. Add green onions, bock choy. Mix well.
- Turn heat down and add in rice noodles
- Mix and serve.

Nutrition per serving: calories: 446 |fat: 2.6g |fiber: 4.8g |protein: 8.1g

3.48 Kidney Bean Pasta Salad

Ingredients

- Half chopped cucumber
- Pasta cooked: 2 cups
- 1 can of kidney beans
- Feta cheese: ¾ cup
- Half cup parsley, fresh
- One spring onion
- Half can sweet corn

Instructions

- In a big bowl, add all ingredients and mix well
- Add light sodium soy sauce on top if you want
- Enjoy

Nutrient per serving: Calories: 160 g| Protein: 14 g| Carbohydrates: 19 g| Fiber: 2 g| Total Fat: 3 g| Sodium: 189 mg| Phosphorus: 88 mg| Potassium: 176 mg|

3.49 Tuna Pasta Salad

Ingredients

- Chopped red onion: 1 cup
- Light tuna: 2 cans, packed in water
- Chopped celery: 1 cup
- Elbow pasta: 3 cups, cooked
- Low-fat mayonnaise: half cup.
- Frozen peas: 1 cup
- Red wine vinegar: 1 tbsp.
- Salt and pepper to taste

Instructions

- Cook pasta as per instructions, without salt, wash under cold water.
- In a bowl, add celery, pasta, peas, onion, tuna, mayonnaise, pepper, salt, and vinegar.
- Mix well and enjoy it.

Nutrition per serving: Calories: 355kcal | Carbohydrates: 59g | Protein: 17g | Fat: 5g | Saturated |fat: 1g | Cholesterol: 11mg | Sodium: 114mg | Potassium: 364mg | Fiber: 4g | Sugar: 5g | Calcium: 56mg | Iron: 2mg

3.50 Healthy Pizza Pasta Salad

Ingredients

- 16 oz. pasta
- ⅔ cup of low sodium Italian dressing
- 1 can chickpeas, drained
- One large green bell pepper, chopped
- One cup of sun-dried tomatoes, julienned
- Dried oregano leaves: 2 tsp

Instructions

- Cook pasta as per instructions, without salt
- In a bowl, add all ingredients, including cooked and washed pasta
- Mix well

Nutrition per serving: Calories: 257 |Fat: 4g |Saturated fat: 0g |Carbohydrates: 50g |Sugar: 6g| Sodium: 359mg |Fiber: 8g| Protein: 8g |Cholesterol: 0mg

3.51 Mediterranean Zucchini Noodle Salad

Ingredients

- Two zucchinis
- 1 onion peeled
- 2 cloves of crushed garlic
- One cup of bock choy quarter
- 1 cup: chickpeas
- Red wine vinegar: 2 tablespoons

- Half cup of crumbled feta cheese
- Olive oil: 1/4 cup
- 1 cup of red bell pepper
- Lemon juice: 1 tablespoon
- Dijon mustard: 1 teaspoon
- Salt and pepper to taste
- Dried oregano: 1 teaspoon

Instructions

- In a big jar, add all ingredients and mix.
- Spiralizer the zucchini.
- Spiralizer half the red onion.
- Mix these two noodles
- Add bock choy, chickpeas, feta cheese in the bowl.
- Add the dressing over vegetables and mix.
- Drizzle the salad dressing over the veggies and gently stir everything together. Serve and enjoy.
- **Nutrient per serving**: Calories: 151 g| Protein: 7.8 g| Carbohydrates: 12.1 g| Fiber: 3.4 g| Total Fat: 2.9 g| Sodium: 103 mg| Phosphorus: 87 mg| Potassium: 92 mg|

Chapter 4: Kidney-Friendly Chicken & Pork Recipes

4.1 Herb-Roasted Chicken Breasts

Ingredients

- One onion
- 4 cups of chicken breasts (boneless and skinless)
- 1–2 cloves of garlic
- Ground black pepper: 1 teaspoon
- Olive oil: ¼ cup
- Garlic & Herb Seasoning: 2 tablespoons (no salt added)

Instructions

- In a bowl, chop garlic, onion, add herb seasoning, olive oil, and pepper.
- Add chicken to this mix, cover with plastic wrap, then chill in the fridge for four hours.
- Let the oven preheat to 350 F
- Place marinated chicken on foil on a baking tray
- Add the marinade over chicken and bake for 20 minutes
- For browning, Broil for five minutes.

Nutrition Per Serving: Calories 270 | total Fat 17 g| Saturated Fat 3 g| Trans Fat 0 g| Cholesterol 83 mg| Sodium 53

mg| Carbohydrates 3 g| Protein 26 g|
Phosphorus 252 mg| Potassium 491
mg| Dietary Fiber 0.6 g| Calcium 17
mg

4.2 Zesty Chicken

Ingredients

- Olive oil: 2 tablespoons

- Balsamic vinegar: 2 tablespoons

- Green onion: 1/4 cup

- Paprika: 1/4 teaspoon

- 8 ounces of chicken breast (skinless and boneless)

- Black pepper: 1/4 teaspoon

- Fresh oregano: 1 teaspoon

- Half teaspoon of garlic powder

Instructions

- In a mug, whisk olive oil and balsamic vinegar. Add chopped green onion, herbs, and seasoning, mix well. Cut chicken into two pieces.

- In a zip lock bag, add chicken and pour marinade over. Let it chill in the fridge for half an hour to 24 hours.

- Grease the pan, cook chicken until chicken's internal temperature reaches 170 F

Nutrients per serving: Calories 280|
Protein 27 g| Carbohydrates 4 g| Fat 16
g| Cholesterol 73 mg| Sodium 68 mg|
Potassium 280 mg| Phosphorus 205
mg| Calcium 26 mg| Fiber 0.3 g

4.3 Slow-Cooked Lemon Chicken

Ingredients

- One pound of chicken breast, skinless, boneless

- Dried oregano: 1 teaspoon

- Chicken broth: ¼ cup, low sodium

- 2 cloves of pressed garlic

- Black pepper: ¼ teaspoon

- Fresh basil: 1 teaspoon, chopped

- Butter: 2 tablespoons, unsalted

- Lemon juice: 1 tablespoon

- Water: ¼ cup

Instructions

- In a bowl, mix black pepper, oregano. Rub this mix on chicken.

- In a skillet, melt butter, brown the chicken in butter, then place in the slow cooker.

- Add garlic, water, broth, and lemon juice in the skillet. Let it boil, then pour over chicken

- Cook on low for five hours, high for two and a half hours.

- Baste chicken and add basil.

- Cover it, cook on high for half an hour minutes.

Nutrition Per Serving: Calories 197 |
Total Fat 9 g| saturated Fat 5 g| Trans
Fat 0 g| Cholesterol 99 mg| sodium 57

mg| carbohydrates 1 g| Protein 26 g| Phosphorus 251 mg| potassium 412 mg| Dietary Fiber 0.3 g| Calcium 20 mg

4.4 Turmeric Lime Chicken

Ingredients

- Vegetable oil: 4-5 TBSP
- Three minced garlic cloves
- Turmeric: one tablespoon
- Cilantro: two tablespoon
- Two beaten egg whites
- Boneless chicken breasts: six (not thick)
- Four halved juicy limes
- Bread crumbs: 2 cups
- Salt and pepper to taste

Instructions

- Make four tiny cuts on top of each chicken breast, then season on both sides with pepper and salt. This scoring will help the marinade flavors absorb the meat quicker and enable the chicken breasts to cook quicker and more evenly.

- In a large bowl, combine fresh lime juice, minced garlic, and chopped cilantro and put the mixture's chicken breasts. Cover it up, and let stay at room temperature for half an hour.

- Whisk the eggs. Combine the turmeric powder and the panko or bread crumbs in another container

- Put each breast of chicken in the beaten egg bowl and switch to cover with egg. Then cover the turmeric/bread crumb mixture on both sides of each chicken breast.

- Pan-fry the chicken breasts in a wide pan, use oil to coat the pan. Around 6-10 minutes per side, if required, after that, clean the pan. Repeat the process with each chicken breast.

- If the chicken is completely cooked. Serve in a sandwich or with a delicious mango salsa, steamed or sautéed vegetables of your choosing.

Nutrition per serving: 326 kcal | Carbohydrates: 20g | Protein: 29g | Fat: 14g | Potassium 181 mg| Phosphorus 102 mg

4.5 Grilled Moroccan Chicken

Ingredients

- Olive oil: one tbsp.
- Chicken breasts: 1 and ½ pound
- Coriander: 1/8 tsp
- Cumin: 2 tsp.
- Sea salt: ¾ tsp.
- Ginger: half tsp.
- Cinnamon: one tsp.
- Turmeric: half tsp.

- Cayenne: optional

- Paprika: one tsp.

- Lemon juice: two tbsp.

Instructions

- Drizzle lemon juice and olive oil all over the chicken

- Mix the salt and spices in a big bowl. evenly coat chicken in spices mixture

- Let it cool in refrigerate for two hours or overnight

- Heat the barbecue grill to a medium to high temperature. Add chicken and leave for around 5 minutes or until you have created grill lines.

- Shift the chicken away from heat and cook for 15-25 minutes on a lower level,

- Remove from flame, and allow to settle before serving or cutting for 5 minutes.

Nutrition per serving: Kcal 204 | Carbohydrates: 20g | Protein: 36g | Fat: 8g | Potassium 162 mg| Phosphorus 103 mg

4.6 Honey Turmeric Chicken

Ingredients

- Honey: 1 and half tbsp.

- Two minced cloves garlic

- Four chicken thighs (skin on but deboned)

- Turmeric powder: 3/4 tsp

- Salt, to taste

- Oil: 1 tablespoon

- One pinch of cayenne pepper

- Soy sauce: one tbsp.

Instructions

- Combine the chicken with the honey, oyster sauce, garlic, turmeric powder, salt, and cayenne pepper, mix well to combine.

- Put the skillet on medium flame, add the oil. Move the chicken to the skillet and fry on both sides until the skin side becomes light brown, crispy at the bottom and wonderfully browned and crispy. Serve hot.

Nutrition Per Serving: Kcal315| Total Fat 45g | Carbohydrates 16g | Protein37g| Potassium 198 mg| Phosphorus121 mg

4.7 One-Pan Roasted Chicken with Turmeric

Ingredients

- Bone-in; skin on chicken: six pieces

- One sweet onion sliced

- Virgin olive oil: half cup

- Orange juice: half cup

- One juice of a lime

- Honey: 3 tbsp.

- Dry white wine: half cup

- Yellow mustard: 2 tablespoon

- Ground turmeric: 3/4 tbsp.

- Ground coriander: one teaspoon

- Sweet paprika: one teaspoon

- Garlic powder: 1 tbsp.

- Two oranges (sliced)

- One lime, thinly sliced

- One fennel bulb (sliced)

- Pepper and salt, to taste

Instructions

- Combine the orange juice, olive oil, lime juice, white wine, honey, and mustard in a big dish.

- Mix the spices in a bowl: paprika, turmeric, coriander, powdered garlic, black pepper, and salt. To the liquid marinade, add approximately half of the spice blend. combine well

- Dry the chicken pieces with a paper towel and season well with the remaining spice mix. Make sure to season under the chicken skins and add some of the spice blends

- In the large bowl of marinade, add the chicken and the remaining ingredients. Mix it well. Cover and refrigerate for almost two hours. After marination, let the oven pre-heat to 475 F.

- Move the chicken to a large baking pan and the marinade and

everything else, so that it is arranged in one layer. Make sure the skin of the chicken faces upwards. Sprinkle with a splash of salt and brown sugar, if needed.

- Roast for almost 45 mints, or until the chicken is completely cooked and the chicken's skin has browned well. The internal temperature of the chicken should be 170 degrees F.

Nutrition Per Serving: Kcal 382|Fat 14g|Protein 35g|Carbohydrate 38g| Potassium 164 mg| Phosphorus 103 mg

4.8 Anti-Inflammatory Chicken Quinoa

Ingredients

- Olive oil divided: 4 tbsp.

- Boneless, skinless chicken breasts: one pound

- Finely chopped red onion: ¼ cup

- Roasted red peppers: 2 cups

- One minced garlic clove

- Paprika: 1 tsp.

- Crushed red pepper: ¼ tsp(optional)

- Cooked quinoa: two cups

- Ground cumin: half tsp.

- Olives, chopped: ¼ cup

- Diced cucumber: one cup

- Almonds: ¼ cup

- Crumbled feta cheese: ¼ cup
- Salt: ¼ teaspoon
- Ground pepper: ¼ teaspoon
- Fresh parsley: 2 tbsp.

Instructions

- In the upper third of the oven, put a rack; let the broiler preheat to heavy. Place foil on a rimmed baking dish.

- Put salt and pepper on the chicken, and put on the prepared baking sheet. Broil it for 14 to 18 min, rotating once, till a thermometer instant-read added in the thickest section registers 165 degrees F. Move the chicken and slice on a cutting board.

- Meanwhile, put two spoons of oil, cumin, peppers, almonds, crushed red pepper in a food processor. Pulse it until creamy

- In a medium dish, mix olives, quinoa, two spoons of oil, and red onion. mix it well

- Divide the quinoa mixture into four bowls and finish with similar quantities of red pepper sauce, cucumber, and tomato to eat. Sprinkle with parsley and feta.

- Enjoy

Nutrition Per Serving: 219 calories| total fat 26.9g |carbohydrates 31.2g |protein 34.1g | Potassium 187 mg| Phosphorus 132 mg

4.9 Chicken& Quinoa Buddha Bowls

Ingredients

- Salt: ¼ tsp.
- Skinless chicken thighs: five boneless pieces' black pepper: half tsp.

Quinoa

- Light chicken broth: 3 cups
- Olive oil: 1 tbsp.
- Quinoa one and ½ cups
- Salt: ¼ tsp.

Italian Dressing

- Cloves of garlic: one large
- Olive oil: 1and ¾ cups
- Red-wine vinegar: ¾ cups
- Dijon mustard: one tbsp.
- Dried basil: 2 tsp.
- Honey: 1 and ½ tbsp.
- Dried oregano: 2 tsp.
- Ground pepper: ½ tsp.
- Water: 5 tbsp.
- Salt: ½ tsp.

Toppings

- 1 Can of chickpeas (15 ounces), rinsed
- Six radishes, sliced
- Toasted seeds /chopped nuts: ¼ cups

- Sprouts: one cup

Instructions

- For chicken preparation: Preheat oven to 425 degrees F. Put the chicken on a baking tray to roast with a half teaspoon of ground pepper and half a teaspoon of salt.

- Roast the chicken for 14 to 16 minutes, until the thickest section by an instant-read thermometer, registers 165 degrees F.

- Slice four thighs cooking quinoa: in a large saucepan, add broth, one tablespoon of oil, and 1/4 teaspoon of salt. Let it simmer on high heat.

- Switch to a boil and mix in the quinoa. Reduce heat and boil for 15 to 20 minutes, until the quinoa and the grains burst have drained all the moisture.

- Remove from heat, cover for 5 minutes, and let it sit. (Reserve two cups for further use.)

- For making dressing: In a mixer, add honey, vinegar, mustard, water, garlic, oregano, basil, pepper, and salt. Pulse till completely combine. Slowly add oil and puree until smooth, while the blender is still running.

- To make bowls: take four bowls and divide three cups worth of quinoa in them. Cover with chickpeas, chicken, and sprouts

scatter with nuts—drizzle dressing of 3/4 cups.

Nutrition Per Serving: 250 calories| total fat 23g |carbohydrates 20.3g | protein 14.4g| Potassium 199 mg| Phosphorus 134 mg

4.10 Skillet Lemon Chicken & Potatoes with Kale

Ingredients

- Chopped tarragon: one tbsp.

- Boneless, skinless chicken thighs: one pound(trimmed)

- Ground pepper: half tsp. Divided

- Olive oil: 3 tbsp.

- Salt: half tsp. divided

- Light chicken broth: half cup

- Baby kale: 6 cups

- One lemon; sliced

- Four cloves of garlic(minced)

- Baby Yukon Gold potatoes: one pound; halved lengthwise(leached)

Instructions

- Let the oven pre-heat till 400 F

- In a large skillet, heat one tbsp. Of oil.

- Sprinkle with 1/4 teaspoon of salt and pepper on chicken. Cook, rotating once, before browning on both sides, a total of about 5 minutes. Move into a tray.

- Add 1/4 tsp. of salt and pepper to the pan with the remaining two teaspoons of oil, with potatoes.

- Cook potatoes, cut-side down, for around 3 minutes, until browned. Add lemon, broth, garlic, and tarragon. Bring the chicken back into the pan.

- Switch the frying pan to the oven.

- Roast, about 15 minutes, before the chicken is completely cooked and the potatoes are soft.

- Stir the kale into the mixture and roast for 3 to 4 minutes until it has wilted.

Nutrition per Serving: 347 Kcal| total fat 19.3g |carbohydrates 25.6g | protein 24.7g | Potassium 171 mg| Phosphorus 151 mg

4.11 Chicken Souvlaki Kebabs with Couscous

Ingredients

- Four minced garlic cloves

- Boneless, skinless chicken: one pound (breast halves, cut into half-inch strips)

- Dry white wine: 1/3 cup

- Lemon juice: ¼ cup

- Wedges of lemon

- Sliced fennel: 1 cup

- Olive oil: 3 tbsp.

- Salt: half tsp.

- Black pepper: ¼ tsp.

- Dried oregano: 2 tsp.

Couscous

- Large pearl couscous: half cup

- Water: 1 cup

- Dried tomatoes: half cup

- Olive oil: 1 tsp.

- Red sweet pepper: ¾ cup

- Chopped red onion: half cup

- Plain Greek yogurt: 1/3 cup

- Chopped cucumber: half cup

- Salt: ¼ tsp.

- Basil leaves: ¼ cup

- Fresh parsley: ¼ cup

- Lemon juice: one tbsp.

- Black pepper: ¼ tsp.

Instructions

- Making kabobs: In a resalable plastic bag, put the chicken and sliced fennel in a baking dish. For marinade, mix the white wine, lemon juice, oil, garlic, oregano, salt, and pepper mix in a cup. Remove the marinade about 1/4 cup, and put aside.

- Pour over the chicken mixture, the remaining marinade. Mix it in the bag. Marinate for 1 and half hours in the refrigerator, turning bag over, once.

- Meanwhile, soak eight 10- to 12- inch wooden skewers in water for half an hour. Drain the chicken and remove fennel and marinade—thread chicken on skewers, accordion-style.

- Grill skewers of chicken, covered, over medium-high heat for eight minutes or until the chicken is no longer pink keep turning 2, 3 times.

- With the reserved 1/4 cup of marinade, brush it on kabobs.

- Preparing the couscous: Pour one teaspoon of olive oil over medium heat in a saucepan. Cook and mix until light brown for about 4 minutes. Then add 1 cup of water. Let it boil on low flame.

- Simmer and cover for ten minutes, until couscous is soft and all the liquid is absorbed, adding the last 5 minutes of half cup snipped dried tomatoes; cool it down. The couscous is moved to a large bowl.

- Stir in the 3/4 cup of chopped red pepper, half cup of each chopped cucumber and chopped red onion, 1/3 cup simple fat-free Greek yogurt, 1/4 of a cup each sliced basil leaves and fresh parsley, one tablespoon of lemon juice, and 1/4 teaspoon of each fresh ground black pepper and salt

- Serve with couscous, lemon wedges, and basil leaves.

Nutrition Per Serving: 332 Kcal|total fat 9.4g |carbohydrates 27 g| protein 32.1g | Potassium 198.9 mg| Phosphorus 112 mg

4.12 Chicken and Snap Peas Stir Fry

Ingredients

- Skinless chicken breast: 1 and ¼ cups (sliced)

- Vegetable oil: 2 tbsp.

- Two minced garlic cloves

- Snap peas: 2 and ½ cups

- Black pepper and salt

- Cilantro: 3 tbsp. and for garnish

- One bunch of scallions (thinly sliced)

- Soy sauce, low sodium: 3 tbsp.

- One red bell pepper(sliced)

- Sriracha: 2 tsp.

- Sesame seeds:2 tbsp.

- Rice vinegar: 2 tbsp.

Instructions

- Heat the oil over medium flame in a large pan. Stir in the garlic and scallions, then sauté for around one minute until fragrant. Stir in the snap peas and bell pepper, then sauté for 2 to 3 minutes until soft.

- Add the chicken and cook for 4 to 5 minutes until golden and thoroughly cooked, and the vegetables are tender.

- Add the sesame seeds, soy sauce, rice vinegar, Sriracha, mix well to blend. Allow boiling the mixture for two minutes.

- Add the cilantro and garnish with coriander and sesame seeds. Serve hot

Nutrition Per serving: 228 calories|11g fat|11g carbs|20g protein| Potassium 210 mg| Phosphorus 105 mg

4.13 Sheet-Pan Chicken Fajita Bowls

Ingredients

- Chicken tenders: 1 and ¼ pounds
- Chili powder: 2 tsp.
- Salt divided: ¾ tsp.
- Chopped steamed kale: 4 cups
- Ground pepper: ¼ tsp.
- Ground garlic: half tsp.
- Smoked paprika: half tsp.
- Ground cumin: 2 tsp.
- Olive oil: 2 tbsp.
- One red bell pepper, sliced
- One Can of black beans(15 ounces)
- Greek yogurt: ¼ cup
- Juice of lemon: 1 tsp.
- One green bell pepper, sliced
- Water: 2 tsp.
- One onion, sliced

Instructions

- Let the oven pre-heat till 425 F
- put the baking sheet in the oven
- in a big bowl, Combine half tsp of salt, chili powder, garlic powder, cumin. Paprika and pepper.
- Transfer 1 teaspoon from a mixture of spices to a small bowl, put it away. Stir one tablespoon of oil into the remaining spice blend.
- Add onion, bell peppers (red and green) to the chicken, stir to mix.
- Remove the pan from the oven cover with oil spray.
- Lay the chicken mixture into the pan in one layer—roast 15 minutes.
- In the meantime, mix the remaining 1/4 tsp of salt, oil with the kale and black beans. In a wide bowl, swirl to coat.
- Remove the frying pan from the oven. Stir the vegetables and chicken spread the beans kale uniformly.
- Roast 5 to 7 minutes more before the chicken is cooked through and the vegetables are ready.

- Add lime juice, water, and yogurt to the rest of the spice blend, mix well

- Take four bowls. Add the vegetables and chicken to bowls.

- Add yogurt dressing and serve hot.

Nutritional Per Serving: 243 calories| total fat 9.9g |carbohydrates 23.7g | protein 42.7g | Potassium 121 mg| Phosphorus 109 mg

4.14 Chicken with Red Bell Pepper Olive, & Feta Topping

Ingredients

- Half of a cup olive oil

- Four, skinless chicken breasts

- Half of a cup lemon juice

- Two tsp. of chopped garlic

- One cup of chopped red bell pepper

- 2 tsp. fresh oregano

- 1/3 of a cup sliced olives

- Black pepper and salt, to taste

- Half of a cup crumbled Feta cheese

Instructions

- Score the chicken breast from the top. But not to cut too far.

- Combine lemon juice, olive oil, oregano, and garlic.

- Take 1/4 cup of the mixture and then put aside

- Put chicken breast into a Ziploc bag and let it marinate in the refrigerator for at least an hour or as long as the whole day.

- Take the chicken out of the fridge when you are about to serve, and let it come to room temperature when cutting the olives and bell pepper.

- Mix the sliced pepper and olives, crumbled Feta, and the remaining marinade.

- Heat one teaspoon olive oil in a skillet over medium flame

- Take the chicken from the marinade and prepare for it to be cooked, scored side down in the skillet.

- Cook each side for about four minutes or completely cooked through

- Season the chicken with salt and black pepper fresh-ground to compare.

- Place chicken over the feta, tomato, and olive, on a platter. serve hot.

Nutrition Per Serving: 243 calories| total fat 9.9g |carbohydrates 23.7g | protein 42.7g | Potassium 129 mg| Phosphorus 98.9 mg

4.15 Roast Chicken with Turmeric & Fennel

Ingredients

- Six pieces of bone-in, skin-on chicken
- Half cup of olive oil
- Half cup of orange juice
- One lime juice
- Half-cup dry white wine
- honey: 3 tablespoon
- One tablespoon of garlic powder
- Yellow mustard: 2 tablespoon
- Turmeric: 3/4 tablespoon powder
- One teaspoon of ground coriander
- One teaspoon of sweet paprika
- One onion: sliced
- Fennel bulb: sliced
- 2 Oranges, peel on, sliced
- Salt and Pepper, to taste
- Lime slices(optional)

Instructions

- To make the marinade combine the white wine, olive oil, orange juice, honey, lime juice, and mustard in a bowl.

- Mix the spices in a small bowl: garlic powder, turmeric, paprika, coriander, pepper, and salt. To the liquid marinade, add approximately half of the spice blend. Mix it well

- With a paper towel, pat the chicken dry and season well with the remaining spice mix, rub the spice mix under the skin.

- In the large bowl of marinade, add the seasoned chicken and the remaining ingredients. cover with plastic wrap and refrigerate for two hours

- Let the oven pre-heat to 475F. Move the chicken to a large baking pan and the marinade and everything else; make sure the chicken's skin faces upwards. Sprinkle with a splash of salt and brown sugar,

- Let it bake for 45 minutes until the chicken is cooked through

- Serve hot

Nutrition per serving: Kcal 243| fat 18 g| Carbs 20.8 g| Protein 22 g| Potassium 150 mg| Phosphorus 111 mg

4.16 Roasted Pork Tenderloin with Vegetables & Quinoa

Ingredients

- Italian Dressing
- Olive oil: 1 and ¾ cup
- Sugar: 1 and ½ tbsp.
- Dried basil: 2 tsp.
- Dijon mustard: 1 tbsp.
- Clove garlic: one large
- Dried oregano: 2 tsp.

- Red-wine vinegar: ¾ cup
- Salt & ground pepper: half tsp. each
- Water: 5 tbsp.

Pork & Vegetables

- Olive oil: 3 tbsp.
- Pork tenderloin: one pound
- Parsnips: 2 medium
- Broccoli crown: 1 medium
- Carrots: four small
- Salt: ¾ tsp.
- Ground pepper: ¾ tsp.
- Italian seasoning: 2 tsp.
- Balsamic glaze: 4 tbsp.
- Quinoa: cooked in chicken broth and cooled

Instructions

- For making dressing: in a mixer, add sugar, vinegar, water, mustard, basil, garlic, oregano, pepper, and salt. Pulse till creamy.
- Slowly add oil and pulse until smooth, while the processor is running. reserve 2 tbsp. of dressing aside
- To cook pork & vegetables: In a wide sealable container, put pork and 1/4 cup of dressing. Take out air and seal rub the sauce all over the pork.
- Keep cool in the refrigerator for as long as you like.

- In the upper and lower thirds of the oven, put racks; let the oven preheat to 425F
- Peel the carrots, then parsnips, then cut into one-inch pieces.
- Cut the broccoli into florets. Add 2 tsp of oil, Italian seasoning, and half tsp. Each and salt and pepper to the vegetables. Place over a broad baking sheet,
- Take out the pork from the marinade and use paper towels to pat dry. Sprinkle the pork with and pepper. Heat one tablespoon of oil over medium flame.
- Add the pork and roast for 3 to 5 minutes, until browned. Switch over the pork and then move the pan to the upper rack. Place the vegetables on the shelf below.
- Roast the pork roughly for 20 minutes with an instant-read thermometer added into the thickest section registers 145 degrees F.
- Roast the vegetables for 20 to 25 minutes, turning once or twice, until soft and browned in patches.
- Move the pork to a clean cutting board, and give 5 minutes to rest. Toss away the vegetables with the remaining two spoons of dressing.
- Slice the pork and serve with the quinoa, grilled vegetables, and over balsamic glaze drizzled.

Nutrition Per Serving: Kcal 490 | total fat 21.7g |carbohydrates 44.3g | protein 31g| Potassium 280 mg| Phosphorus 205 mg

4.17 Grilled Lemon Herb Chicken Salad

Ingredients

Lemon-Herb Chicken

- Boneless, chicken breasts: 6 cups(skinless)
- Chopped fresh dill: 1 tablespoon
- Extra-virgin olive oil: 3 tablespoons
- Chopped fresh oregano: 1 tablespoon
- Kosher salt and freshly ground black pepper
- Juice of 2 lemons, and zest
- Chopped fresh parsley: 3 tablespoons

Salad

- Chicken broth: 2 and a ½ cups
- Barley: 1 cup
- Juice of 1 lemon and zest
- ⅓ of a cup extra-virgin olive oil
- One halved red onion, thinly sliced
- mustard: 1 tablespoon
- 2 heads of red-leaf lettuce, diced
- Dried oregano: 1 teaspoon
- Kosher salt and freshly ground black pepper

Instructions

- To make Lemon Herb Chicken Put the chicken inside a large plastic sealed plastic bag. In a bowl, add lemon juice, olive oil, dill, lemon zest, parsley, and oregano and mix well.

- Then pour this marinade into the sealed bag, seal, and chill for almost half an hour.

- To make the salad: in the meantime, put the chicken broth and barley over medium flame in a saucepan and let it simmer.

- Cover the pot and steam until the barley is soft for almost 30-45 minutes. Drain and set it aside.

- Mix the oregano lemon juice, lemon zest, and mustard in a bowl, then slowly drizzle in the olive oil and mix properly. Add salt and pepper to taste.

- Let your grill pre-heat at high. Take chicken out from marinade and sprinkle with freshly ground black pepper and salt.

- Grill chicken on each side until charred and completely cooked through, cook for almost ten minutes, flipping as required, take the chicken from the grill and set it aside.

- In a big bowl, mix the onion, and lettuce, drizzle the dressing and coat well.

- Cut the chicken into slices, and serve

Nutrition per serving: 309 calories|15g fat |4g carbs|31g protein| Potassium 134 mg| Phosphorus 121 mg

4.18 Greek Chicken & Rice Skillet

Ingredients

- Green olives: 1 cup
- 6 pieces of chicken thighs
- Chicken broth: 2 and a ½ cups
- Long-grain rice: 1 cup
- Dried oregano: 1 teaspoon
- Garlic powder: 1 teaspoon
- Three lemons
- Extra-virgin olive oil: 2 tablespoons
- Half red onion, chopped
- 2 cloves of minced garlic
- ⅓ of a cup fresh chopped fresh parsley
- Chopped fresh oregano: 1 tablespoon (more for garnishing)
- Kosher salt and freshly ground black pepper

Instructions

- Let the oven pre-heat to 375°F.
- Add salt and pepper to chicken thighs, adjust the seasoning. mix garlic powder, dried oregano, zest of one lemon in a small mixing bowl, rub this mixture on chicken thighs generously
- In a wide skillet, heat the olive oil over medium flame. Put the meat, skin side down, then sear for nine minutes until the meat turns light brown. Move to the plate and set aside.
- Add the garlic and onion in the pan, and sauté for around five minutes until opaque. Add the rice and sauté for one minute; then season with salt.
- Add the broth and let it boil then slow to simmer. Add the zest and lemon juice, oregano. Cut two slices for later.
- Put the chicken skin side down into the rice. Put the skillet to pre-heated oven till all the broth is absorbed, and chicken is thoroughly cooked, for almost 25 minutes.
- Now turn the broiler, and put the lemon slices on the chicken. Broil until the lemons are finely crispy, and the chicken skin is also crispy, flor almost three minutes.
- Then add the olives over the lemon slices, top with parsley leaves, and serve hot.

Nutrition per serving: 703 calories|34 g fat|32 g carbs|38g protein| Potassium 183 mg| Phosphorus 111 mg

4.19 Pesto Chicken Salad

Ingredients

- Packed coarsely chopped arugula: One cup
- Half of a cup nonfat plain Greek yogurt
- Lemon juice: 2 teaspoons
- Half of a teaspoon salt
- ⅓ of a cup mayonnaise
- Chopped or shredded cooked chicken: 3 cups
- Half of a cup cherry tomatoes halved
- Pesto: 2 tablespoons
- Toasted pine nuts: 3 tablespoons
- Half of a teaspoon freshly ground black pepper
- Minced shallot: 2 tablespoons

Instructions

- In a big mixing bowl, add yogurt, shallot, mayonnaise, freshly ground black pepper, salt pesto, and lemon juice.
- Then add in the chicken, tomatoes, and arugula.
- Garnish with pine nuts.
- Chill in refrigerator until cold for two hours. Or serve at room temperature.

Nutrition per serving: 209 calories| total fat 15.7g |carbohydrates 3.4g | protein 13g

4.20 Edamame & Chicken Greek Salad

Ingredients

- One and half cups of frozen shelled edamame thawed
- Boneless skinless(trimmed)chicken breast: one piece
- ¼ of a cup red-wine vinegar
- Chopped romaine: 8 cups
- ¼ of a cup sliced red onion
- Extra-virgin olive oil: 3 tablespoons
- ¼ of a teaspoon salt
- Half of a European cucumber, sliced
- Half of a cup crumbled feta cheese
- ¼ of a cup sliced fresh basil
- ¼ of a teaspoon freshly ground black pepper

Instructions

- In a large saucepan, add chicken and add cover it by water by 2 inches. Let it boil. Lower the heat and let it simmer and cook. Check with an instant-read thermometer add into the chicken. It should show 165 degrees F after cooking for 15 minutes.
- Move the chicken to a clean cutting surface and cool it for five minutes. With a fork, shred it, or chop into pieces.
- In the meantime, add kosher salt, freshly ground black pepper, vinegar, oil in a big mixing bowl. Then Add romaine,

edamame, feta, onion, cucumber, basil, and the chicken. Toss well.

- Serve right away.

Nutrition per serving: 336 calories| total fat 21.6g |carbohydrates 14.2g |protein 22.3g| Potassium 111 mg| Phosphorus 78 mg

4.21 One Pot Greek Chicken and Lemon Rice

Ingredients

- Chicken marinade
- Lemon juice: 4 tbsp.
- Five pieces of chicken thighs, bone-in, skin-on: one kg
- Zest of 2 lemons
- 4 cloves of minced garlic
- Half tsp of kosher salt
- Dried oregano: 1 tbsp.

Rice

- Chicken broth or stock: 1 and half cups
- Olive oil: 1 and half tbsp. separated
- Long-grain rice: 1 cup, uncooked
- Freshly ground Black pepper
- 3/4 of a cup water
- Dried oregano: 1 tbsp.
- One small onion, finely chopped
- ¾ of a tsp kosher salt

For Garnish

- Finely chopped parsley or oregano
- Lemon zest should be fresh

Instructions

- In a reseal able plastic bag, add the chicken and marinade ingredients and mix well. Set it aside for 20 minutes, for the minimum or preferably overnight.
- Let the oven preheat to 350°F.
- Heat half tbsp. Of olive oil over medium-high heat in a deep skillet.
- Put the chicken skin side down, cook till golden brown, and then flip and cook on the other side. Take chicken out from skillet and set it aside.
- Clean the skillet and put skillet again on the flame.
- Heat one tbsp. of extra virgin olive oil over medium flame in the skillet. Add onion and cook until transparent, for three minutes.
- Add the remaining ingredients for Rice and the Marinade reserve.
- Let the liquid boil and then let it simmer for 30 seconds.
- Put the chicken on top of the rice, then cover the skillet. Let it bake for 35 minutes after removing the cover and bake for another ten minutes, or until all the

moisture is absorbed and the rice is soft.

- Remove from the oven and, if necessary, allow to rest for ten minutes before serving, garnished with oregano parsley and fresh lemon zest.

Nutrition per serving: Calories 323|fat 21g|carbs 33g|protein 18g| Potassium 220 mg| Phosphorus 105 mg

4.22 Greek Cauliflower Rice Bowls with Grilled Chicken

Ingredients

- Boneless, skinless: 4 cups of chicken breasts
- Cauliflower rice: 4 cups
- Extra-virgin olive oil: 7 tablespoons divided
- ⅓ of cup diced red onion
- Feta cheese(crumbled) :2 tablespoons
- Half cup of sliced fresh dill, divided
- Lemon juice: 3 tablespoons
- Oregano: 1 teaspoon (dried)
- ¾ of teaspoon kosher salt, divided
- Diced cucumber: One cup
- For garnish Lemon wedges
- Half teaspoon freshly ground black pepper, divided

Instructions

- Let the grill preheat on high.

- In a wide skillet over medium flame, add extra virgin olive oil (two tbsp.), add 1/4 teaspoon of salt, cauliflower, and onion. Stir often and let it cook. Cauliflower will become tender after cooking for five minutes. Turn off the heat and add 1/4 cup of dill. Set it aside.

- Rub one tbsp. of olive oil all over the chicken. Add 1/4 teaspoon of freshly ground black pepper and 1/4 teaspoon of salt over chicken.

- Grill it for about 15 minutes, and add an instant-read thermometer into the thickest part of the chicken should read 165 degrees F.

- Then, in a medium mixing bowl, add four tablespoons of oil, oregano, lemon juice, and 1/4 teaspoon of each salt and pepper and mix well.

- In four serving bowls, add cauliflower rice and add chicken slices, feta, cucumber, and 1/4 cup of dill.

- Garnish with lemon wedges, serve right away and enjoy.

Nutrition per serving: 411 calories| total fat 27.5g |carbohydrates 19.5g |protein 29g| Potassium 145 mg| Phosphorus 106 mg

4.23 Zucchini Noodles with Pesto & Chicken

Ingredients

- Boneless, skinless: 4 cups of chicken breast, cut into bite-size pieces
- 1/4 cup extra-virgin olive oil and two tablespoons more
- Four pieces of trimmed medium-large zucchini
- ¼ of cup shredded Parmesan cheese
- Fresh basil (packed) leaves: 2 cups
- Lemon juice: 2 tablespoons
- One large clove of chopped garlic
- ¼ of cup toasted pine nuts
- Half teaspoon of freshly ground black pepper
- ¾ of teaspoon kosher salt, divided

Instructions

- Cut the zucchini in length into big, thin strands, utilizing a spiral vegetable slicer. Chops these long noodles so the strands would not be very long. Put the zucchini in a colander, and add 1/4 teaspoon of salt. Let it drain for almost half an hour, then press gently to extract any remaining moisture.

- In a food processor bowl, add Parmesan, basil, 1/4 teaspoon of salt, pine nuts, 1/4 cup of olive oil, black pepper, lemon juice, and garlic, and pulse on high until smooth

- Put a wide skillet over medium flame, add one tbsp. of oil. Add chicken in an even layer then add 1/4 teaspoon of salt.

- Let it cook, often stirring, for about 5 minutes. Then Transfer to a bowl and stir in three tablespoons of the pesto.

- To the pan, add the remaining one tablespoon of olive oil. Then Add the dried zucchini noodles mix carefully for two-three minutes.

- Add these noodles to the bowl with the cooked chicken. Add the leftover pesto and toss lightly to coat.

Nutrition per serving: 430 calories| total fat 31.6g | carbohydrates 9.4g |fiber 2.5g |protein 28.6g| Potassium 187 mg| Phosphorus 143 mg

4.24 Slow Cooker Mediterranean Chicken

Ingredients

- Boneless skinless chicken breasts: 4 pieces' medium to large
- Kosher salt, to taste
- Freshly ground black pepper, To taste
- Italian seasoning: 3 teaspoons
- Juice of one large lemon: 2 tablespoons approx.
- Minced garlic: one tbsp.
- One medium onion, diced

- Roasted red peppers: 1 cup (roughly chopped)
- Capers: 2 tablespoons
- Fresh basil, thyme, and oregano for garnish

Instructions

- Put a wide skillet over medium flame, add chicken seasoned with salt and ground black pepper, and cook for two minutes. Both sides will be browned. Then add chicken to the slow cooker. Make sure to grease it before adding chicken.

- Add red peppers, capers, and onions to slow cooker. Put them on the side of chicken, not over chicken.

- In the meanwhile, mix lemon juice, garlic, and Italian seasoning. Pout it all over the chicken.

- Cover it and cook for two hours on high and four hours on low.

- Garnish with oregano, fresh thyme, and basil.

- Serve right away and enjoy.

Nutrition per serving: 304 calories| total fat 20.9g |carbohydrates 23.6g | |protein 19.9g| Potassium 187 mg| Phosphorus 121 mg

4.25 Spiced Pan-Roasted Chicken with Olives, Figs, and Mint

Ingredients

- Chicken broth: 1 cup

- Chicken: one whole
- Ground coriander: 1 tablespoon
- ⅛ of a teaspoon cayenne
- Fresh lemon juice: 2 tablespoons
- Kosher or sea salt: 1 tablespoon
- Eight figs: dried, roughly diced
- Extra-virgin olive oil: ¼ cup
- ¼ of teaspoon ground cinnamon
- Roughly chopped green olives: 2 tablespoons (roughly diced)
- Chopped mint: 1 tablespoon, extra more for garnish

Instructions

- Remove the backbone of chicken with kitchen shears and flatten with your hands

- In a mixing bowl, add coriander, salt, two tablespoons of olive oil, cayenne, and cinnamon.

- Rub this spice blend all over the chicken and put the chicken skin side up in the fridge, do not cover, for 4-24 hours.

- Let the oven pre-heat to 400F.

- To an oven-safe sauté pan add two tablespoons of olive oil and heat over medium flame until hot. Then add chicken. It should be skin side down and cook until golden brown.

- Put in the preheated oven, and cook for half an hour.

- Flip the chicken, then add mint, lemon juice, both types of olives, chicken broth, and figs to the oven-safe pan and let it cook in the oven for an hour an hour more internal temperature with instant-read thermometer reaches 165°.

- When chicken is cooked through, top with thinly sliced mint.

- Transfer the chicken to a clean surface and cut in slices

- To a serving plate, put the chicken and put pan drizzling on top, garnish with olives, figs mix.

- Serve right away and enjoy.

Nutrition per serving: 501 calories| total fat 36g| protein 34g.| carbs 23 g| Potassium 145 mg| Phosphorus 102 mg

4.26 Chicken Caprese Sandwich

Ingredients

- Extra virgin olive oil: 4 tablespoons, or more, divided

- Half lemon juiced

- ¼ cup of sliced fresh basil leaves

- Kosher salt and freshly ground black pepper

- One log of fresh mozzarella cheese of8 ounces, sliced into rounds (1/4 thickness)

- Skinless: 2 pieces of boneless chicken breasts

- Fresh parsley: 1 teaspoon(sliced)

- One loaf of ten ounces, sourdough bread, cut in half lengthwise

- Balsamic glaze or balsamic vinegar, to taste

Instructions

- In a big mixing bowl, add parsley, black pepper, two tablespoons of extra virgin olive oil, salt, lemon juice, mix it well. Pour this over chicken breasts and toss lightly to coat well and let the chicken rest at room temperature.

- Put a grilling pan over medium heat. Add the chicken breast to the grilling pan, without the marinade, and add black pepper and salt. Flip the chicken after four minutes.

- Cook for three minutes more, till grill marks, appear.

- Lower the flame, and cover the chicken and cook till the instant-read thermometer reads 185 degrees.

- Turn off the heat and slice the chicken, and set it aside.

- Pour one tablespoon of extra-virgin olive oil to each side of the bread and grill it until golden brown.

- Slice the bread into three slices for each half. Add 3-4 slices of chicken, few slices of mozzarella cheese to each slice. Pour balsamic vinegar, extra virgin olive oil on top. Add basil leaves on top.

- Season with more salt and black pepper.

- Serve hot

Nutrition per serving: calories 321 g| Fat 32.06g|Carbohydrates 46.88g|Protein 34.42g| Potassium 210 mg| Phosphorus 125 mg

4.27 Smothered Pork Chops & Sautéed Greens

Ingredients

Smothered Pork Chops

- Flour: 1 cup + 2 tablespoons
- Six pork loin chops
- Paprika: 2 teaspoons
- Half cup of olive oil
- Onion powder: 2 teaspoons
- Half cup fresh scallions
- Black pepper: 1 tablespoon
- Garlic powder: 2 teaspoons
- Beef stock, low-sodium: 2 cups
- 1 and a half cups of sliced onions

Sautéed Greens

- Unsalted butter: 1 tablespoon

- Fresh collard greens: 8 cups, blanched and chopped
- Onions: ¼ cup, diced
- Garlic: 1 tablespoon, diced
- Black pepper: 1 teaspoon
- Crushed red pepper flakes: 1 teaspoon
- Olive oil: 2 tablespoons

Instructions

- Let the oven preheat to 350° F.

- For Pork Chops, Mix onion powder, black pepper, garlic powder, and paprika. Rub half of the mixture on both sides of the pork chops and combine the other half with one cup of flour.

- Coat the pork chops with the flour mix

- In a Dutch oven, heat oil on medium-high

- Brown the pork chops for 2 to 4 minutes on every side.

- Take out from pan and reserve two tbsp. Of oil,

- Sauté onions 4–6 minutes or until translucent. Add in two tbsp. of flour and mix with onion for one minute

- Gradually add the stock and mix until thickened.

- Add pork chops to the pan and coat with sauce. Cover with foil and cook in the oven at 350° F for 30-45 minutes.

- Take out from the oven and let rest for ten minutes

- For Sautéed Greens, In a pan, melt butter on medium-high heat. Add garlic and onions for 4 to 6 minutes

- Add greens and sprinkle with red pepper and black and cook for 5 to 8 minutes on high flame. Keep mixing.

- Serve right away

  Nutrition per serving: Cal 464|fat 28g|cholesterol 71 mg| protein 27 g| phosphorous 289 mg| potassium 604 mg

4.28 One-Pot Chicken & Dumplings

Ingredients

- Parsley: 1 tablespoon

- Cold unsalted butter: 5 tablespoons, divided

- One stalk of celery sliced

- Two carrots, diced

- One onion, minced

- All-purpose flour: 1 and 1/4 cup, divided

- Diced cooked chicken: 1 to 2 cups

- Green beans: 1/3 pound, cut into one-inch pieces

- Half tsp of thyme

- One bay leaf

- Chicken broth, low sodium: 3 cups

- Celery seed: 1/4 tsp

- Half tsp of rosemary

- Baking powder substitute: 1 teaspoon

- Three drops of sriracha sauce

- Pepper to taste

- Half cup of almond milk

- Chopped parsley: 2 tablespoons

Instructions

- In a pan, melt three tbsp. of butter sauté carrots, onion, and celery, cook until translucent for four minutes.

- Add 1/4 cup of flour cook for one minute. Add broth, keep mixing, let it boil, lower the heat and simmer for five minutes. Add in spices, chicken, and green beans.

- Take 2 tablespoons parsley, baking powder, one cup of flour, ½ tsp. of salt(optional), add two tbsp. of butter, almond milk mix.

- Add this mixture to the chicken, cover it, and let it simmer for 12 minutes.

- Serve right away

Nutrients Per Serving: Calories 230| Total Fat 10.3g| Cholesterol 27.1mg| Sodium 145.8mg| Total Carbohydrate 30.2g| Dietary Fiber 4.3g| Protein 5.2g|

Iron 2.6mg| Potassium 455.3mg| Phosphorus 226.6mg

4.29 Easy Crispy Lemon Chicken

Ingredients

- Herb seasoning blend: 1 teaspoon
- Cooked white rice: 4 cups
- Half cup of all-purpose white flour
- One-pound chicken breasts (skinless and boneless), cut into slices
- Black pepper: 1/4 teaspoon
- One large egg white
- Salt: 1/4 teaspoon
- Half cup of lemon juice
- Water: 2 teaspoons
- Olive oil: 2 tablespoons

Instructions

- Season the chicken with herbs, pepper, and salt.
- In a bowl, whisk the egg white with water
- Coat chicken in egg white mix then in flour.
- Fry chicken in olive oil until light brown, but do not overcook the chicken
- Add lemon juice on top and serve.

Nutrients per serving: Calories 316| protein 22 g| Carbohydrates 39 g| Fat 8 g| Cholesterol 82 mg| sodium 144 mg| Potassium 234 mg| Phosphorus 201 mg| Calcium 28 mg| Fiber 0.8 g

4.30 Grilled Pineapple Chicken

Ingredients

- Chicken breast: 1-1/4 pound, skinless and bone-in
- Dry sherry: 1 cup
- Soy sauce, reduced-sodium: 1 tablespoon
- Four rings of pineapple
- Pineapple juice: 1 cup

Instructions

- In a zip lock bag, add all ingredients except for pineapple.
- Marinate it overnight in the refrigerator.
- Grill the marinated chicken for 15-20 minutes until cooked.
- In the last few minutes of cooking, grill pineapple for two minutes on each side. Serve with chicken breast.

Nutrients per serving: Calories 211| Protein 26 g| Carbohydrates 20 g| Fat 3 g| Cholesterol 67 mg| Sodium 215 mg| Potassium 376 mg| Phosphorus 198 mg| Calcium 21 mg| Fiber 0.5 g

4.31 Sheet Pan Chicken with Green Beans & Cauliflower

Ingredients

- One and 1/3 cups of frozen green beans
- Cauliflower floret: one and a half cups
- 2 cups of chicken strips, raw
- Italian dressing: 1 tablespoon
- Olive oil: 1 teaspoon
- Unsalted butter: 4 tablespoons

Instructions

- Let the oven preheat to 400° F.
- Toss cauliflower in one tsp. of olive oil.
- Spray a baking tray with cooking spray.
- Add the strips of chicken on 1/3 of the tray. Place the cauliflower down on the other 1/3 of the pan. Add frozen beans to the tray also.
- Melt butter and pour over the cauliflower, green beans, and chicken. Add Italian seasoning over all the tray.
- Bake for 20-30 minutes. Check them after 20 minutes and serve.

Nutrients per serving: Calories 330| Protein 25 g| Carbohydrates 19 g| Fat 17 g| Cholesterol 102 mg| Sodium 308 mg| Potassium 545 mg| Phosphorus 280 mg| Calcium 47 mg| Fiber 2.5 g

4.32 Pulled Pork

Ingredients

- Oil: 1 tablespoon
- One cup of minced onion
- 3 cloves of minced garlic
- 4 pounds of pork shoulder roast (boneless), cut in cubes, trimmed fat
- Worcestershire sauce: 2 and a half tablespoons
- Ketchup: half cup, no salt added
- Honey: 3 tablespoons
- Red wine vinegar: 3 tablespoons
- Liquid smoke: 1 teaspoon
- Half teaspoon of black pepper
- Orange-flavored drink, sugar-free: 1 cup

Instructions

- In a skillet in oil, cook onion, garlic, and pork for five minutes. Keep stirring.
- Add the rest of the ingredients and mix well. Let it boil, then simmer on low flame while being covered for one hour.
- Uncover it and cook for half an hour, till the liquid has evaporated.
- Shred the pork with two forks. Serve.

Nutrients per serving: Calories 233| Protein 22 g| Carbohydrates 7 g| Fat 13 g| Cholesterol 77 mg| Sodium 104 mg| Potassium 365 mg| phosphorus 197 mg| Calcium 21 mg| Fiber 0.1 g

4.33 Roast Pork with Apples

Ingredients

- Tart apple: 5 cups, sliced and peeled
- 3-pound of boneless, trimmed pork loin roast
- One slice of diced maple bacon
- Cider vinegar: 2 tablespoons
- Onion: 2 cups, chopped
- Black pepper: 1/4 teaspoon
- Green cabbage: 3 cups, sliced
- Four carrots, cut into large chunks
- Dry white wine: 3/4 cup
- Maple syrup: 2 tablespoons

Instructions

- Let the oven preheat to 375° F.
- In a Dutch oven, spray with cooking spray over medium-high heat, cook pork for 15 minutes, brown it on all sides. Take the pork out.
- Add bacon and onion to the pan, sauté for five minutes, or until tender.
- Add the pork to the pan, then add carrots, apples, and cabbage, the rest of the ingredients, let it simmer. Put the pan in the oven.
- Cook uncovered for 45 minutes at 375 F
- Turn the pork over, cook for half an hour.
- The internal temperature of pork should be 155° F.

Nutrients per serving: Calories 244| Protein 30 g| Carbohydrates 13 g| Fat 8 g| Cholesterol 68 mg| Sodium 99 mg| Potassium 538 mg| Phosphorus 185 mg| Calcium 48 mg| Fiber 3.1 g

4.34 Lemon Rosemary Pork

Ingredients

- Chicken broth, low-sodium: 1/4 cup
- All-purpose white flour: 2 tablespoons
- 1 pound of pork cutlets
- Half teaspoon of pepper
- Olive oil: 2 teaspoons
- Fresh rosemary: 1 tablespoon, chopped
- One cup lemon juice

Instructions

- In a zip lock bag, mix pepper and flour. Add pork and coat well
- Heat oil, cook pork for 2-3 minutes, on each side over medium-high heat.
- It should not be pink in the middle. Check with a sharp knife.
- Take out in plate keep warm with foil.
- In a skillet, add chicken broth, rosemary, and lemon juice. Let it boil for 3-4 minutes.

- Pour sauce over pork and serve.

Nutrients per serving: Calories 228| Protein 24 g| Carbohydrates 8 g| Fat 10 g| Cholesterol 69 mg| Sodium 51 mg| Potassium 378 mg| Phosphorus 160 mg| Calcium 18 mg| Fiber 0.5 g

4.35 Baked Pork Chops

Ingredients

- Unsalted margarine: 2 tablespoons
- Half cup of all-purpose flour
- Water: 1/4 cup
- Cornflake crumbs: 3/4 cup
- One large egg white
- Six pork chops: center cut
- Salt: 1/4 teaspoon
- Paprika: 1 teaspoon

Instructions

- Let the oven preheat to 350 °F.
- In a bowl, add flour.
- In a bowl, whisk water and egg. Add cornflake crumbs to another plate
- Coat pork chops in flour, then in egg, then in cornflakes.
- Put pork on a baking sheet, spray with oil, pour melted margarine
- Season with salt and paprika, chill in the fridge for one hour or more.

- Bake for 40 minutes or until cooked.
- Serve.

Nutrients per serving: Calories 282| Protein 23 g| carbohydrates 25 g| Fat 10 g| Cholesterol 95 mg| Sodium 263 mg| Potassium 394 mg| Phosphorus 203 mg| Calcium 28 mg| Fiber 1.4 g

4.36 Pork Fajitas

Ingredients

- Dried oregano: 1 teaspoon
- One green bell pepper, sliced
- One onion, sliced
- Pineapple juice: 2 tablespoons
- 2 cloves of garlic
- 4 flour tortillas
- Olive oil: 1 tablespoon
- Boneless pork: 1 pound, lean, cut into strips
- Half teaspoon of cumin
- Hot pepper sauce: 1/4 teaspoon
- 2 tbsp. of vinegar

Instructions

- In a big zip lock bag, add pineapple juice, hot sauce, oregano, vinegar, garlic, and cumin. Add pork into it and marinate for 10-15 minutes
- Let the oven preheat to 325° F.
- Heat the tortillas in foil.

- In a skillet, sauté green pepper, onion, pork in oil until pork is no longer pink for five minutes
- Serve with warm tortillas.

Nutrients per serving: Calories 406| Protein 26 g| Carbohydrates 34 g| Fat 18 g| cholesterol 64 mg| Sodium 376 mg| Potassium 483 mg| Phosphorus 267 mg| Calcium 57 mg| Fiber 2.4 g

4.37 Herb-Rubbed Pork Tenderloin

Ingredients

- One and a half tablespoons vegetable oil
- Dried rosemary: 1 teaspoon
- Dried parsley: 1 teaspoon
- Dried thyme: 1 teaspoon
- 2 cloves of minced garlic
- Dried basil: 1 teaspoon
- Black pepper: 2 teaspoons
- 2 pork tenderloins
- Dijon mustard: 2 tablespoons

Instructions

- In a bowl, add spices, garlic, mustard, mix well.
- Rub this mix over tenderloins—marinade for two hours.
- Let the oven preheat to 400° F.
- In a skillet in oil, brown the tenderloins, then place it on a baking dish.

- Bake t for 20 minutes or until the meat thermometer shows 160° F.
- Let it rest for 10-15 minutes before serving.

Nutrients per serving: Calories 178| Protein 24 g| Carbohydrates 1 g| Fat 8 g| Cholesterol 67 mg| Sodium 160 mg| Potassium 401 mg| Phosphorus 230 mg| Calcium 20 mg| Fiber 0.4 g

4.38 Dumplings Divine

Ingredients

Filling

- Ginger: 1 Tbsp., chopped
- 2 cups of ground pork
- Soy sauce, low-sodium: 2 Tbsp.
- Cabbage: 1 cup, thinly sliced
- Dough
- All-purpose flour: 2 cups
- Water: 3/4 cup

Sauce

- Balsamic vinegar: 1 Tbsp.
- Green onion: 1 Tbsp.
- Olive oil: 1 Tbsp.

Instructions

- To prepare the filling, mix pork, cabbage, ginger, and soy sauce. Keep in the fridge.
- In another bowl, mix flour with water. Knead until dough forms.

- Make one inch balls from the dough, flatten them and add one tbsp. of filling.
- Seal the edges with water. Pinch them as you like.
- In a large pot, boil the water and add dumplings. Cook for 10 to 15 minutes. And serve with sauce

Nutrients per serving: (5 dumplings): Cal 310| Total Fat 17.2g| Cholesterol 52.4mg| Sodium 142.8mg| Total Carbohydrate 20.5g| Dietary Fiber 0.9g|Protein 16.9g| Iron 2.1mg| Potassium 411.3mg| Phosphorus 196.2mg

4.39 Sweet N' Sour Meatballs

- 1.5 cups of chopped vegetables
- 8 cups of ground meat pork
- 1/4 tsp of nutmeg
- 2 cups of cooked rice
- Low sodium soy sauce: 1 Tbsp.
- Worcestershire sauce, low sodium: 1 Tbsp.
- 1/4 cup of unsweetened almond milk
- 2 tsp of garlic powder
- Half cup of finely diced onion

Sweet and Sour Sauce
- Pineapple juice: 2 cups
- Soy sauce, reduced-sodium: 2 tablespoons
- Half tsp sesame seed oil
- Vinegar: 1/3 cup
- Cornstarch: 6 tablespoons
- 5 cups of pineapple chunks, canned
- Water: 2/3 cup
- Honey: half and a little more cup

Instructions
- Let the oven preheat to 375° F.
- Chop the vegetables.
- Mix chopped vegetables, meat, rice, pepper, garlic powder, soy sauce, Worcestershire sauce, nutmeg. Mix well. Do not over mix.
- Make one inch balls and put them on a baking sheet
- Bake for 10-15 minutes.
- Pour the juice out of pineapple cans, add water in the juice to make two cups.
- Mix starch with sesame seed oil, honey, pineapple juice, soy sauce, water, and vinegar.
- Heat until becomes thick, mix constantly. Turn off the heat.
- Add pineapple chunks, bell peppers, meatballs, and sauce, heat on low until serving time.

Nutrient per serving (2 meatballs): Calories: 123 g| Protein 11.2 g| Carbohydrates: 15.3 g| Fiber: 1.8 g| Total Fat: 3 g| Sodium: 105 mg| Phosphorus: 78 mg| Potassium: 77 mg| 3

4.40 Honey-Garlic Low Sodium Marinated Kebabs

Ingredients

- Bragg's Liquid Amino: 1/4 cup
- 1/4 cup of olive oil
- 3 cloves of crushed garlic cloves
- Four medium chicken breast cut into cubes
- 1/3 cup of honey
- Four small onions, cut into cubes
- Black pepper: 1/4 tsp
- Three peppers, cut into cubes

Instructions

- In a zip lock bag, add all ingredients except for onion, peppers.
- Marinate for half an hour or more (overnight)
- Add on skewers alternate with pepper and onion.
- Grill until done.

Nutrients per serving: Calories 143| Total Fat 2.1g| Cholesterol 41.4mg | Sodium 137.4mg| Total Carbohydrate 17.9g| Dietary Fiber 1.4g| Protein 13.9g| Iron 0.5mg| Potassium 447.7mg| Phosphorus 145.5mg

4.41 Hawaiian-Style Slow-Cooked Pulled Pork

Ingredients

- Half teaspoon of garlic powder
- 4 pounds of pork roast
- Half teaspoon of paprika
- 2 tablespoons of liquid smoke
- Onion powder: 1 teaspoon
- Half teaspoon of black pepper

Instructions

- In a bowl, add garlic powder, black pepper, onion, and paprika.
- Run this spice mix on pork. Add pork in a slow cooker. Add liquid smoke
- Add water to half of the slow cooker. Cook on high for 4 to 5 hours.
- Shred with fork and serve

Nutrition Per Serving: Calories 285 | total Fat 21 g| Saturated Fat 7 g| Trans Fat 0 g| Cholesterol 83 mg| Sodium 54 mg| Carbohydrates 1 g| Protein 20 g| Phosphorus 230 mg| Potassium 380 mg| Dietary Fiber 0 g| Calcium 9 mg

4.42 Spicy Grilled Pork Chops with Peach Glaze

Ingredients

- Smoked paprika: 1 teaspoon
- 8 pork chops, center-cut
- Cilantro: 2 tablespoons
- Lime juice: ¼ cup
- Peach preserves: 1 cup
- Zest of one lime
- Half teaspoon of black pepper
- Dried onion flakes: 2 teaspoons

- Soy sauce, low-sodium: 1 tablespoon
- Half teaspoon of red pepper flakes
- Olive oil: ¼ cup

Instructions

- Heat the grill on high.
- In a bowl, add all ingredients except for pork chops, mix well.
- Take out a quarter of the mix and add the rest of it in a zip lock bag with pork chops overnight.
- Grill them for 6 to 8 minutes on each side.
- Glaze with reserved mix and serve.

Nutrition Per Serving: Calories 357 | Total Fat 18 g| Saturated Fat 5 g| trans Fat 0 g| Cholesterol 64 mg| Sodium 158 mg| Carbohydrates 27 g| Protein 23 g| Phosphorus 188 mg| Potassium 363 mg| Calcium 40 mg

4.43 Slow-Cooked Cranberry Pork Roast

Ingredients

- One cup of diced cranberries
- Ground cloves: ⅛ teaspoon
- Brown sugar: 1 tablespoon
- 4 pounds of center-cut pork roast
- Black pepper: 1 teaspoon
- Honey: ¼ cup

- Nutmeg: ⅛ teaspoon
- Zest of orange peel: 1 teaspoon
- Half teaspoon of salt

Instructions

- Season pork roast with pepper and salt. Put in a slow cooker.
- Mix remaining ingredients and pour over the pork.
- Cook on low for 8 to 10 hours.
- Take out from cooker, slice it, and serve with dipping.

Nutrition Per Serving: Calories 287 | Total Fat 14 g| Saturated Fat 5 g| Trans Fat 0 g| Cholesterol 85 mg| Sodium 190 mg| Carbohydrates 8 g| Protein 30 g| Phosphorus 240 mg| Potassium 406 mg| Dietary Fiber 0.4 g| Calcium 40 mg

4.44 Herb-Crusted Pork Loin

Ingredients

- One pork loin roast, boneless
- Fennel seed: 2 tablespoons
- Low sodium soy sauce: 2 tablespoons
- Caraway seed: 2 tablespoons
- Dill seed: 2 tablespoons
- Anise seed: 2 tablespoons

Instructions

- Pour soy sauce on roast and coat well.

- In a baking pan, mix fennel, dill seed, caraway, and anise seed. Coat the pork in this mixture.

- Pack foil around pork and refrigerate for at least two hours or more

- Let the oven preheat to 325 F.

- Remove foil, put pork's fat side up on a rack in a shallow pan, and bake for 35 to 40 minutes each pound. Until the meat thermometer reads 145 F.

- Let rest for three minutes. Slice and serve

Nutrition Per Serving: Calories 224 | Total Fat 13 g| Saturated Fat 5 g| Trans Fat 0 g| Cholesterol 70 mg| Sodium 134 mg| Carbohydrates 2 g| Protein 24 g| Phosphorus 225 mg| Potassium 405 mg| Dietary Fiber 1.0 g| Calcium 53 mg

4.45 Roast Pork Loin with Sweet and Tart Apple Stuffing

Ingredients

- Marmalade Cherry Glaze:

- Half cup of orange marmalade, sugar-free

- Cinnamon: 1/8 teaspoon

- ¼ cup of apple juice

- Nutmeg: 1/8 teaspoon

- ¼ cup of dried cherries

Apple Stuffing

- Half cup of chicken stock, low-sodium

- Canola oil: 2 tablespoons

- Half cup of diced honey crisp apple

- Unsalted butter: 2 tablespoons

- Cubed Hawaiian rolls: 2 cups packed

- Chopped onions: 2 tablespoons

- Fresh thyme: 1 tablespoon

- Chopped celery: 2 tablespoons

- Black pepper: 1 teaspoon

Roast pork loin

- One pound of pork loin, boneless

- Butcher twine: 2 pieces

Instructions

- In a pan, combine all ingredients on medium flame until all is melted and well combined, bring it to simmer. Turn off the heat.

- Let the oven preheat to 400 F

- In a pan, fry all ingredients in oil, do not add chicken stock for 2 to 3 minutes.

- Gradually add a stick until it's only moist, not wet.

- Turn off the heat and let it come to room temperature.

- Cut slits, lengthwise, of one inch in pork, like pockets.

- Add two tbsp. of stuffing to every pocket.

- Tie the pork with twine so that stuffing will remain in place.

- Put the rest of the stuffing on the baking tray, put tied pork on stuffing.
- Bake at 400 F for 45 mints, or until internal temperature is 160 F
- Drizzle over the glaze shut the oven off, and let it rest for 10 to 15 minutes.

Nutrition Per Serving: Calories 263 | Total Fat 14 g| Saturated Fat 4 g| Trans Fat 0 g| Cholesterol 50 mg| Sodium 137 mg| Carbohydrates 22 g| Protein 14 g| Phosphorus 154 mg| Potassium 275 mg| Dietary Fiber 1 g| Calcium 68 mg

4.46 Kidney-Friendly Chicken Salad

Ingredients

- Onion: 1/4, diced
- Half cup of chicken breasts, skinless and boneless
- Spicy brown mustard: 1/4 teaspoon
- One celery stalk, diced
- Half teaspoon of vinegar
- Miracle whip: 1 tablespoon
- Half tsp. of garlic powder

Instructions

- Boil the chicken.
- Shred the cooled chicken
- Add mustard, whip, onions, vinegar, onion powder, celery and mix well.

- Serve.

Nutrient per serving: Calories: 198 g| Protein: 15.3 g| Carbohydrates: 15.4 g| Fiber: 1.9 g| Total Fat: 3.1 g| Sodium: 222 mg| Phosphorus: 101 mg| Potassium: 121 mg|

4.47 Honey Garlic Chicken

Ingredients

- Half cup of honey
- 4 pound of roasting chicken
- Garlic powder: 1 teaspoon
- Olive oil: 1 tablespoon
- Half teaspoon of black pepper

Instructions

- let the oven preheat to 350 F.
- Add olive oil to the pan.
- Add chicken in pan, do not overlap. Coat chicken with all the ingredients
- Bake for one hour or until done. Flip halfway through.
- Serve.

Nutrients per serving: Calories 279 kcals| Sodium 40 mg| Protein 13 g| Potassium 144 mg| Fat 10 g| Calcium 11 mg| carbohydrates 36 g| Phosphorus 99 mg| Fiber 0 g| Cholesterol 40mg

4.48 Seasoned Pork Chops

Ingredients

- 4 lean pork chops fat trimmed
- Vegetable oil: 2 tablespoons
- Black pepper: 1 teaspoon

- Half teaspoon of thyme
- Half teaspoon of sage
- All-purpose flour: ¼ cup

Instructions

- Let the oven preheat to 350°f.
- Add oil to baking pan.
- Mix sage, flour, thyme, and black pepper.
- Coat pork chops in flour mix and place in the pan.
- Bake for 40 minutes, or until cooked
- Serve hot.

Nutrition per serving: 434 calories| 60 mg sodium|19 g protein |79 mg cholesterol |332 mg potassium| 34 g total fat| 12 g carbohydrate |199 mg phosphorus| 10 g saturated fat |35 mg calcium

4.49 Homemade Pan Sausage

Ingredients

- Granulated sugar: 2 teaspoons
- 1 pound of fresh lean ground pork
- Ground black pepper: 1 teaspoon
- Half teaspoon of ground red pepper
- Ground sage: 2 teaspoons

Instructions

- Mix all ingredients to make sausage.

- Make patties of mixture 2 tbsp. each.
- Fry in oil and serve.

Nutritional per serving: 96 calories | 22 mg sodium|6 grams' protein| 43 mg cholesterol |87 mg potassium| 7 grams' total fat| 1-gram carbohydrate |53 mg phosphorus| 2 grams saturated | fiber 72 mg calcium

4.50 Salisbury Steak

Ingredients

- Vegetable oil: 1 tablespoon
- 1 pound of ground pork
- Half cup of diced green pepper
- 1 egg white
- Black pepper: 1 teaspoon
- One diced onion
- Corn starch: 1 tablespoon
- Half cup of water

Instructions

- In a bowl, add green pepper, meat, egg, onion, and black pepper.
- Make patties
- Cook patties in a pan until cooked completely
- Add water and simmer for 15 minutes. Take patties out
- Add the rest of the water, mix with corn starch, let it simmer to thicken.
- Serve the patties with gravy

Nutrition per serving: 249 calories| 128 mg sodium|22 grams' protein| 149 mg cholesterol |366 mg potassium| 57 grams' total fat| 7 grams' carbohydrate| 218 mg phosphorus|3 grams saturated fat| 1-gram fiber| 33 mg calcium

4.51 Jalapeno Pepper Chicken

Ingredients

- Chicken: 2-3 pounds, cut up skinless
- Vegetable oil: 3 tablespoons
- One onion, cut into rings
- 1 and a half cups of chicken stock, low-sodium
- Jalapeño peppers: 2 teaspoons, chopped without seeds
- Half teaspoon of ground nutmeg
- Black pepper: ¼ teaspoon

Instructions

- Brown chicken pieces in oil set it aside
- Sauté onion and add the stock, let it boil.
- Take chicken back to the pan, add pepper and nutmeg. Cover it and simmer for 35 minutes.
- Add in jalapeño peppers.

Nutrition per serving: 143 calories | 45 mg sodium|17 grams' protein| 46 mg cholesterol| 160 mg potassium|7 grams' total fat| 2 grams' carbohydrate |127 mg phosphorus|1 gram saturated fat| 12 mg calcium

Chapter 5: Kidney-Friendly Beef & Turkey Recipes

5.1 Rice with Beef

Ingredients

- 1 cup diced onion
- Vegetable oil: 2 tablespoons
- Rice: 2 cups, cooked
- Half teaspoon sage
- 1 and a half tsp. Seasoning of chili con carne powder
- Black pepper: ⅛ teaspoon
- 4 cups of lean ground beef

Instructions

- Sauté onion and brown the meat in the skillet
- Add seasoning and rice, mix well.
- Turn off the heat and cover it.
- Let it rest for ten minutes, then serve.

Nutrition per serving: 360 calories |1 g trans-fat |78 mg sodium| 23 g protein| 65 mg cholesterol |427 mg potassium|14 g total fat |26 g carbohydrate| 233 mg phosphorus|4 g saturated fat| 2 g fiber| 34 mg calcium

5.2 Cilantro Burger

Ingredients

- Cilantro: 3 tablespoon
- 4 cups of lean ground turkey

- Oregano: ¼ teaspoon
- Black pepper: ¼ teaspoon
- Ground thyme: ¼ teaspoon
- Lemon juice: 1 tablespoon

Instructions

- In a bowl, mix all ingredients.
- Make into patties.
- Fry on a lightly greased skillet and broil for 10 to 15 minutes. Turning halfway once

Nutrition per serving: 171 calories |0 g trans-fat |108 mg sodium|20 g protein |90 mg cholesterol| 289 mg potassium|10 g total fat |0 g carbohydrate |180 mg phosphorus|3 g saturated |fat 0 g| fiber 21 mg calcium

5.3 Borscht

Ingredients

- Cubed beets: 1 and ½ cups(steamed)
- Olive oil: 2 tbsp.
- Light beef broth/vegetable broth: 2 cups
- One onion, diced
- Half teaspoon of salt
- ¼ tsp. of black pepper
- One potato, chopped, leached
- Red-wine vinegar: 2 tsp.
- Fresh parsley
- Sour cream: ¼ cup

Instructions

- Pour the oil on medium flame in a big saucepan. Add onion and fry for four minutes before browning starts.
- Add stock, potato, pepper, and salt; carry to a boil. Lower the heat to a simmer, let it cover, and cook for eight minutes until it is soft.
- Add vinegar and beets go to boil again. Cover and cook until the broth is red, and the potato is tender for almost three minutes.
- In a dish, mix the sour cream. Top the soup with the sour cream blend. enjoy

Nutrition per Serving: 160 calories| total fat 9g |carbohydrates 17.1g |fiber 2.4g |protein 3.7g

5.4 Turkey Apple Breakfast Hash

Ingredients

For(meat)

- Salt to taste
- Minced Turkey: 1 lb.
- Dried thyme: ½ teaspoon
- Cinnamon: ½ teaspoon
- Olive oil: 1 tbsp.

For(hash)

- Cubed frozen butternut squash: 2 cups
- Kale: 2 cups
- Carrots: ½ cup shredded

- Olive oil: 1 tablespoon
- One small onion
- One large zucchini
- Powdered ginger: ¾ teaspoon
- One apple chopped
- Cinnamon: 1 teaspoon
- Turmeric: ½ teaspoon
- Dried thyme: ½ teaspoon
- Salt to taste
- Garlic powder: ½ teaspoon

Instructions

- Heat a tablespoon of oil over medium flame in a skillet. Add turkey and stir until brown. Season with cinnamon, thyme, and sea salt. Set aside.

- Add remaining oil into the same skillet and sauté onion until softened for 2-3 minutes.

- Add the carrots, zucchini, frozen squash, and apple—Cook for around 4-5 minutes, or until veggies soften.

- Add and mix in kale until wilted.

- Add cooked turkey, seasoning, salt and remove from heat, and serve.

Nutrition Per serving: Kcal 156| Fat: 14g| Net Carbs: 13g| Protein: 15.5g

5.5 Baked Turkey Meatballs

Ingredients

- One egg beat
- Minced turkey: 1 pound
- Grated Parmesan cheese: ½ cup
- Fresh breadcrumbs: ½ cup
- Chopped parsley: 1 tablespoon
- Milk: 2-3 tablespoons
- Chopped fresh basil: ½ tablespoon
- Pinch of grated nutmeg
- Chopped oregano: ½ tablespoon

Instructions

- Let the oven pre-heat to 350F.

- Put parchment paper on two baking sheets.

- In a big bowl, add the turkey, breadcrumbs, cheese, herbs, egg, nutmeg, cinnamon, pepper, and milk. The amount of milk you can use needs to be changed depending on how dry your bread. The mixture should be moist that it binds together.

- Roll parts of the meat into roughly 1-inch balls using a teaspoon and put them onto a baking sheet. You should finish off with 25-30 meatballs.

- Bake the meatballs for around 30 minutes, frequently rotating, causing the meat to be cooked through and brown gently.

Nutrition per serving: Cal 216|Fat 3g|Sodium 17mg|Protein 22g|Carbohydrates 32g

5.6 Goat Cheese Pizza

Ingredients

- Olive oil: 1 tsp.
- Turkey breast (one ounce) shredded
- Whole wheat pizza crust: 7 inches -one piece
- Roma tomato: one(sliced)
- Kale: 1 cup
- Crumbled goat cheese:1/4 cup
- Snipped fresh basil: 2 tbsp.
- Red onion: ¼ cup thinly sliced

Instructions

- Take one spoonful of olive oil and brush it on the pizza crust.
- Add chicken breast, kale, turkey tomato, goat cheese, and red onion. Bake according to the Instructions on the crust package.
- For serving, sprinkle with basil.

Nutrition Per Serving: 219 calories| total fat 10g | carbohydrates 23g |protein 14g.

5.7 White Turkey Chili with green beans

Ingredients

- Chicken broth: 4 cups
- Ground turkey: 1 pound
- One onion, diced
- Four minced garlic cloves
- Olive oil: 2 tbsp.
- One cup of small cut beans
- Ground cumin: 2 tsp.
- White beans: one and a half cups
- Cayenne pepper: 1 tsp.
- Salt pepper, to taste
- Ground coriander: 1 tsp.

Instructions

- Heat the olive oil in a big pot over low flame. Stir in the onion and sauté for 6 to 8 minutes until translucent. Add the garlic and proceed to cook for one minute, until fragrant.
- Stir in the turkey and cook for 5 to 7 minutes until browned and thoroughly cooked. Stir in the coriander, cumin, and cayenne pepper. Add salt and pepper, and cook for two minutes until fragrant.
- Add the broth. Bring the soup over medium flame to a boil. Reduce heat to low and simmer for half an hour, until tastes develop
- Add the beans and cook for three minutes.
- Spoon the chili in bowls and finish with two teaspoons of green beans. Serve hot.

Nutrition Per serving: 144 calories|14g fat|22g carbs|21g protein

5.8 Greek Turkey Burgers with Tzatziki Sauce

Ingredients

Turkey Burgers

- One pound minced turkey
- Olive oil: one tbsp.
- Half cup parsley
- Two minced garlic cloves
- One large egg
- One minced sweet onion
- Half teaspoon of dried oregano
- Bread crumbs: ¾ cup
- Salt & pepper to taste
- Half teaspoon of red chili flakes

Tzatziki Sauce

- One tbsp. of olive oil
- Half cucumber, diced
- ¼ cup of parsley
- 2 tbsp. of lemon juice
- One cup of Greek yogurt
- Garlic powder: 1 pinch
- Pepper and salt, to taste

Burger Topping

- Half onion, sliced
- Four whole-wheat buns
- Lettuce leaves
- Six slices of tomatoes

Instructions

- Heat olive oil over medium flame in a skillet. Add the onion and fry, for 3 to 4 minutes, until translucent. Add the garlic and sauté for one minute more, until fragrant. set it aside
- Mix the cooled onion mixture with the egg, parsley, oregano, red-pepper flakes with ground turkey in a bowl. Add the crumbs, season with pepper and salt, and whisk until combined.
- Let the oven Preheat to 375 ° F.
- Form four modest size patties of the meat mixture. spray oil on a skillet and place it on medium flame
- Put the burgers in the skillet and fry for five minutes per side until golden brown. Move the skillet to the oven and cook for fifteen more minutes till the burgers are thoroughly cooked.
- Sauce: In a medium dish, mix the cucumber with yogurt, add the olive oil, garlic powder, and lemon juice.
- Using salt and pepper to season, then whisk in the parsley.
- Topping: Put each burger on the bottom half of a bun and cover it with around 1/4 cup of tzatziki sauce, two leaves of lettuce, two slices of tomatoes, and the top half of the bun. Serve hot.

Nutrients per serving: 226 calories|14g fat|22g carbs|27g protein

5.9 Ground Turkey Sweet Potato Stuffed Peppers

Ingredients

- 2 cups of minced turkey
- Two minced cloves of garlic
- Half cup of chopped onions
- One tbsp. of olive oil
- Half of a cup tomato sauce, no salt added
- One and 2/3 cups of diced sweet potatoes, leached
- Two cuts in half, bell peppers
- Salt and pepper, to taste
- Red chili flakes (optional)
- Parsley

Instructions

- Let the oven pre-heat till 350F
- Heat the olive oil in a skillet over medium flame.
- Place the turkey and garlic in the skillet. Stir from time to time, and cook for around 10 minutes or until the meat is brown. break any lumps of meat
- Stir in the onions and cook until light brown.
- Put the sweet potatoes on top, cover the pan, and cook until soft. It takes about eight minutes to finish.
- Add the chili flakes, tomato sauce, pepper, and salt. Add more olive oil or a bit of water if needed to cook the potatoes.
- Grease the pan and arrange the peppers. inner side up
- Add the ground turkey-sweet potato mixture in each half of the bell pepper.
- Bake for around half an hour uncovered, or until the peppers are soft, take out from the oven, then garnish with parsley.

Nutrition per serving: Kcal 324| Fat: 13.9g| Saturated Fat: 4.4g, |Carbohydrates: 25.6g|Protein: 26.3g

5.10 Mediterranean Bento Lunch

Ingredients

- One pita bread(whole-wheat) quartered
- 1 and a half cup of grilled turkey breast tenderloin
- ¼ of a cup rinsed chickpeas
- ¼ of a cup chopped tomato
- Chopped olives: 1 tablespoon
- Grapes: one cup
- ¼ of a cup chopped cucumber
- Chopped fresh parsley: 1 tablespoon
- Extra-virgin olive oil: half teaspoon
- Red-wine vinegar: 1 teaspoon
- Hummus: 2 tablespoons

Instructions

- In a mixing bowl, add tomato, feta, cucumber, olives, vinegar, oil, chickpeas, and parsley and toss well until well combined.

- Put this mixture in a dish.

- Put turkey or chicken (if using) in another dish.

- Add pita, hummus, and grapes side by side in small containers.

- Serve all these together in a lunch box or a box with different containers.

- Pack it away and enjoy it later.

Nutrition per serving: 497 calories| total fat 13.8g |carbohydrates 60.5g |protein 36.7g

5.11 Turkey Meatball Soup

Ingredients

- 4 cups of lean ground turkey

- Bread: 2 slices

- Kale: 4 cups

- ¼ of a cup of almond milk

- 2 cloves of garlic pressed

- One medium shallot finely diced

- ½ of a teaspoon freshly grated nutmeg

- One teaspoon of oregano

- 1/4 of a teaspoon red pepper flakes

- Italian parsley chopped: 2 tablespoons

- 2 carrots cut into slices

- One egg beat

- One tablespoon of olive oil

- Chicken or vegetable broth: 8 cups

- One can of 15- ounce white Northern beans rinsed, drained

- Half yellow onion finely diced

- Kosher salt and freshly ground pepper

Instructions

- In a large mixing bowl, add milk, cut the bread into pieces, and let it soak in milk. Add the garlic, turkey, nutmeg, shallot, red pepper flakes, salt, oregano, pepper, egg, cheese, and parsley. Mix carefully with your hands. Use a scooper to make half-inch balls.

- Put a wide skillet on medium flame, heat the olive oil, then sear the meatballs gently on every side for two minutes. Turn off the heat and set it aside.

- Add the onion, stock, beans, kale, and carrots to a 5 to 7 quarter slow cooker.

- Add meatballs the kale, and cook for four hours at low or until the meatballs start floating to the top.

- Garnish the soup with Parmesan grated cheese, red pepper flakes, and fresh leaves of parsley.

Nutrition per serving: 250 calories|
total fat 23g |carbohydrates 20.3g | pro-
tein 14.4g

5.12 Steak & Onion Sandwich

Ingredients

- Vegetable oil: 1 tablespoon
- Four chopped steaks
- Italian seasoning: 1 tablespoon
- Black pepper: 1 tablespoon
- 4 sliced rolls
- Lemon juice:1 tablespoon
- One onion, sliced in rings

Instructions

- In a bowl, mix meat with Italian seasoning, black pepper, and lemon juice
- In a pan, brown the steaks until tender over medium flame.
- Turn the heat down, add onions, cook until tender.
- Serve on a sliced bread roll with onion rings.

Nutrition per serving:345 calories |
247 mg sodium|14 g protein| 40 mg
cholesterol |200 mg potassium|21 g to-
tal fat |26 g carbohydrate |115 mg
phosphorus|7 g saturated fat |2 g fi-
ber | 98 mg calcium

5.13 Taco Stuffing

Ingredients

- Half tsp. of Tabasco sauce
- Vegetable oil: 2 tablespoon
- Italian seasoning: 1 teaspoon
- Lean ground beef: 1 and ¼ pounds
- Half tsp. Of teaspoon black pepper
- Garlic powder: 1 teaspoon
- Half tsp. Of ground red pepper
- Onion powder: 1 teaspoon
- One medium taco shells
- Half head of shredded lettuce
- Half tsp. of nutmeg

Instructions

- In a skillet, add all ingredients except lettuce and taco. Cook until well mixed.
- Add cooked meat in taco shells with shredded lettuce.

Nutrition per serving: 176 calories
|124 mg sodium|14 g protein| 56 mg
cholesterol| 258 mg potassium|9 g total
fat| 9 g carbohydrate |150 mg phospho-
rus |2 g saturated fat |0 g fiber |33 mg
calcium

5.14 Stuffed Green Peppers

Ingredients

- Vegetable oil: 2 tablespoon
- 2 cups of ground lean beef or turkey
- Onions: ¼ cup, Diced
- Celery: ¼ cup, Diced
- Lemon juice: 2 tablespoons
- Celery seed: 1 tablespoon

- Italian seasoning: 2 tablespoons
- Black pepper: 1 teaspoon
- Half tsp. Of honey
- Paprika
- 1 and a half cups of cooked rice
- Six small green peppers, seeds removed

Instructions

- Let the oven preheat to 325 F
- Sauté celery, meat, and onion, until meat is brown
- Add rest of the ingredients, do not add paprika green peppers.
- Mix well and turn off the heat
- Add the mixture into peppers. Wrap with foil and place in a dish.
- Bake for half an hour.
- Sprinkle with paprika and serve.

Nutrition per serving: 131 calories | 36 mg sodium|9 g protein |28 mg cholesterol |160 mg potassium|4 g total fat |15 g carbohydrate |83 mg phosphorus|1 gram saturated fat| 1-gram fiber |38 mg calcium

5.15 Curried Turkey & Rice

Ingredients

- Cooked white rice: 2 cups
- Vegetable oil: 1 teaspoon
- Chicken broth, low-sodium: 1 cup
- One diced onion

- Unsalted margarine: 1 tablespoon
- 1-pound of turkey breast, cut into cutlets
- Curry powder: 2 teaspoons
- Honey: 1 teaspoon
- Flour: 2 tablespoon
- Half cup of non-dairy creamer

Instructions

- In a skillet, cook the turkey for ten minutes, until no longer pink.
- Turn off the heat and keep warm on another plate.
- In the same skillet, add margarine, curry powder, and onion. Stir for five minutes. Then add flour, mixing continuously
- Add in honey, creamer, and broth. Mix until it becomes thick.
- Add turkey back to skillet— Cook for two minutes.
- Serve with rice.

Nutrient per serving: Calories 154 |Sodium 27 mg| Protein 8 g| Potassium 156 mg| Fat 5 g| calcium 25 mg| Carbohydrates 20 g| Phosphorus 88 mg| fiber 1 g| Cholesterol 14 mg

5.16 Tasty Beef Ribs

Ingredients

- Chili powder: 2 teaspoons
- 4 pounds of large beef ribs

- Paprika: 1 tablespoon
- Half tsp. Of garlic powder
- Pineapple juice: 1/4 cup
- Red pepper: 1/8 teaspoon
- Mustard powder: 1/4 teaspoon

Instructions

- In roasting pan, put ribs, meat side down in racks, roast for half an hour at 450 F. drain it
- Pour pineapple juice on ribs.
- Mix the rest of the ingredients, and sprinkle on ribs.
- Turn the temperature to 350 F. then roast for 45 to 60 minutes, with meat side up.

Nutrient per rib: Calories 187 kcals| Sodium 41 mg| Protein 19 g| Potassium 233 mg| Fat 11 g| Calcium 11 mg| carbohydrates 2 g| Phosphorus 149 mg| Cholesterol 56 mg

5.17 Roasted Turkey

Ingredients

- Poultry seasoning: 1 teaspoon
- 12-pound turkey
- Four sprigs of sage
- Turkey stock, low-sodium: 1 cup
- Four sprigs of rosemary
- Half cup of unsalted butter
- Four sprigs of parsley
- Four sprigs of thyme

Instructions

- Let the oven preheat to 425 F.
- look at the cooking time on the plastic wrapping of the turkey.
- Clean the turkey cavity of the giblet, neck. Rinse the turkey and pat dry
- Loosen the skin around drumsticks and breast with fingers.
- Rub seasoning on turkey under the skin.
- Add rosemary, parsley, thyme, sage between flesh and turkey skin.
- Insert a thermometer in the fleshy part.
- Drench turkey in melted butter, place in roasting pan breast side up.
- Cover with aluminum foil, loosely.
- Cook for half an hour, then turn the temperature to 325° F.
- Baste turkey after 15-20 minutes with stock and pan liquid.
- In the last half, an hour remove foil. Cook for 3-4 hours until the meat thermometer shows 165 F.
- Let it rest for half an hour before slicing.

Nutrients per serving: Calories 144| Protein 25 g| Carbohydrates 0 g| Fat 4 g| Cholesterol 64 mg| Sodium 57 mg| Potassium 256 mg| Phosphorus 182 mg| Calcium 22 mg

5.18 Turkey Vegetable Chili

Ingredients

- Cayenne pepper: 1/4 teaspoon
- Olive oil: 1 tablespoon
- Half cup of chopped onion
- 2 cloves of garlic minced
- 1-pound of lean ground turkey
- Diced zucchini: 2 cups
- Chili powder: 2 teaspoon
- Paprika: 1 and a half teaspoons
- 14 ounces of tomatoes canned, crushed, no salt added
- Black pepper: 1/4 teaspoon
- Ground cumin: 1 and a half teaspoons

Instructions

- Sauté the onion, turkey, zucchini, and garlic until tender.
- Drain the excess fluids. Add spices and tomatoes. Cover it and simmer for 30 minutes

Nutrients per serving: Calories 164| Protein 17 g| Carbohydrates 6 g| Fat 8 g| Cholesterol 47 mg| sodium 214 mg| Potassium 517 mg| Phosphorus 189 mg| Calcium 56 mg| Fiber 2.0 g

5.19 Mama's Meatloaf

Ingredients

- Low-fat mayonnaise: 2 tablespoons
- One egg whisked
- Half cup of bread crumbs
- 1-pound lean ground turkey

Seasonings

- Worcestershire sauce, low-sodium: 1 tablespoon
- Garlic powder: 1 teaspoon
- Beef Bouillon: 1 teaspoon low sodium
- Half teaspoon of red pepper flakes
- Onion powder: 1 teaspoon

Instructions

- Let the oven preheat to 375° F.
- In a bowl, add all ingredients, do not add the meat, mix until well combined.
- Add the meat and mix.
- Add meat to meatloaf pan. Cover with the foil—Bake for 20 minutes.
- Remove the aluminum foil and cook for five minutes.
- Turn off the oven, let it rest for ten minutes before serving.

Nutrition Per Serving: Calories 367 | Total Fat 23 g| Saturated Fat 8 g| Trans Fat 1 g| cholesterol 127 mg| sodium 332 mg| carbohydrates 14 g| Protein 25 g| Phosphorus 273 mg| Potassium 460 mg| Dietary Fiber 0.7 g| Calcium 32 mg

5.20 Turkey Soup

Ingredients

- 1 potato, diced(leached)
- 1 cup ground turkey
- 1 teaspoon cayenne pepper
- 1 onion, diced
- 1 tablespoon olive oil
- ¼ carrot, diced
- 2 cups of water

Instructions

- In a saucepan, heat the olive oil and add the chopped onion and carrot.

- For 3 minutes, prepare the vegetables. Then stir them well and add the cayenne pepper and ground turkey.

- Add the diced potato and stir well with the spices. Cook them for an extra 2 minutes.

- Add water, Cover the lid and simmer for 20 minutes to make the broth.

Nutrients Per serving: 317 calories|31.8g protein|14.2g carbohydrates| 16.9g fat| 2.3g fiber|112mg cholesterol| 131mg sodium| 319mg potassium.

5.21 Turkey Bolognese with Zucchini Noodles

Ingredients

- 2 tbsp. of Olive Oil
- 1 lb. of ground turkey
- one Onion, chopped
- Four Zucchini, spiralized
- Chicken stock: 4 cups, no salt added
- Red bell peppers, chopped: 1 cup
- Garlic Cloves Minced: 2 tbsp.
- Half tsp of Red Pepper Flakes
- Cayenne: 1/4 tsp
- 1/4 lb. of Spaghetti
- Nutmeg: 1/4 tsp
- Ground Bay Leaves: 1/4 tsp
- One tsp. of Oregano
- Dried Basil: 1/4 cup

Instructions

- In a pan, sauté onion, turkey, garlic until meat is browned.

- Add stock and all herbs and seasoning (do not add basil), bell peppers. Let it simmer for almost two hours.

- Cook pasta as per instructions, and add zucchini noodles halfway through.

- Add olive oil to pasta so it won't stick.

- When almost all the liquid is absorbed, add basil and noodles. Cook for 2 to 3 minutes, and serve

Nutrients per serving: Cal 212 |calcium 59 mg| potassium 253 mg| phosphorous 249 mg| protein 19 g| carbs 24 g

5.22 Turkey Gravy

Ingredients

- Pan juices of turkey: 1 cup
- Turkey fat: 4 tablespoons, pan drippings
- Giblet stock: 2 cups
- All-purpose white flour: 4 tablespoons
- Half teaspoon of salt

Instructions

- In a saucepan, heat the fat. Add in flour, whisk and let it boil.
- Add pan juices, salt, and stock.
- Keep mixing until it thickens. Lower the heat and simmer for ten minutes.

Nutrients per serving: Calories 87| Protein 2 g| Carbohydrates 4 g| Fat 7 g| Cholesterol 25 mg| Sodium 146 mg| Potassium 43 mg| Phosphorus 19 mg| Calcium 6 mg

5.23 Easy Turkey Sloppy Joes

Ingredients

- One and a half pounds of ground turkey with less fat
- Half cup of red onion, chopped
- Grilling Blend seasoning: 1 tablespoon
- Honey: 2 tablespoons
- Half cup of green bell pepper, chopped
- Tomato sauce, low-sodium: 1 cup
- Worcestershire sauce, low sodium: 1 tablespoon
- Six buns

Instructions

- In a skillet, cook turkey over medium flame until cooked through. Don't drain
- In a bowl, mix all seasoning with tomato sauce.
- Add seasoning mix to turkey. Turn the heat low and cook for ten minutes.
- Place in buns and serve.

Nutrients per serving: Calories 290| protein 24 g| Carbohydrates 28 g| Fat 9 g| cholesterol 58 mg| Sodium 288 mg| Potassium 513 mg| Phosphorus 237 mg| calcium 86 mg| Fiber 1.8 g

5.24 Roasted Turkey Breast with Salt-free Herb Seasoning

Ingredients

- Three pounds of half turkey breast, with skin and bone-in
- 1/4 cup of butter
- 1/4 cup of onion, minced
- Herb seasoning blend, salt-free: 1 tablespoon

Instructions

- Let the oven preheat to 350° F.
- Melt butter, sauté onion with herb seasoning blend.

- Separate the mixture into two bowls.

- In a roasting pan, put turkey breast skin side down. Add one tbsp. of seasoning and coat it.

- Turn over turkey and loosen skin. Add three tbsp. of seasoning between skin and flesh. Secure with toothpicks.

- Put in the oven and cook for 60 minutes.

- Take out from the oven and spread the rest of the seasoning over the turkey's skin.

- Cook for 15-20 minutes, until the thermometer, inserted reads 160° F.

- Rest the turkey breast for 10 to 15 minutes before serving.

Nutrients per serving: Calories 203| Protein 25 g| carbohydrates 1 g| Fat 11 g| Cholesterol 76 mg| Sodium 88 mg| Potassium 265 mg| Phosphorus 184 mg| Calcium 20 mg| Fiber 0 g

5.25 Turkey and Beef Meatballs

Ingredients

- one egg

- 1 pound of ground chuck beef

- Onion & Herb seasoning: 1 tablespoon

- Soft bread crumbs: 1 cup

- 1 pound of ground turkey

- Ground pepper: 1 teaspoon

- Worcestershire sauce, low sodium: 1 teaspoon

- Half cup of beef broth, reduced-sodium

- Dried parsley: 1 tablespoon

Instructions

- Let the oven preheat to 350° F.

- Add parchment paper on two baking sheets

- In a big bowl, mix both meats with dry ingredients, set it aside

- In another bowl, combine egg, broth, and low sodium Worcestershire sauce

- To the meat, add the wet ingredients. Mix well.

- Make one-inch meatballs and put on a baking sheet

- Bake for half an hour, turning halfway through.

- Serve hot with sauce

Nutrients per serving: Calories 175| Protein 16 g| Carbohydrates 3 g| Fat 11 g| Cholesterol 69 mg| Sodium 120 mg| potassium 236 mg| Phosphorus 142 mg| calcium 18 mg| Fiber 0.1 g

5.26 Turkey Bowtie Pasta

Ingredients

Pasta

- One sliced red pepper

- Cooked bowtie pasta: 4 cups

- Diced zucchini: 1 cup

- Black pepper
- Raw mushrooms: 1 cup
- 1 lb. of ground turkey

Sauce

- White flour: 4 tbsp.
- Margarine: 5 tbsp.
- Hot water: 2 cups
- Lemon juice: 1 tsp
- 1 tsp any seasoning no salt added
- Garlic powder: 1 tsp
- 1/4 tsp of red pepper flakes
- Sour cream: 4 tbsp.

Instructions

- In a pan, melt margarine, add flour, and mix. Slowly add hot water.
- Add sour cream and mix well, then add red pepper flakes, seasoning, lemon juice, garlic powder, mix for 1 to 3 minutes. Turn off heat and mix until cools slightly
- Cook the turkey in a pan sauté mushroom and zucchini till tender. Add peppers but do not soften them. Add black pepper, pasta, sauce, and turkey to vegetable mix well.

Nutrient per serving: Calories 516 g| Protein: 28 g| Carbohydrates: 43 g| Fiber: 3 g| Total Fat: 25 g| Sodium: 257 mg| Phosphorus: 257 mg| Potassium: 430 mg

5.27 Lime Grilled Turkey

Ingredients

- ⅔ lb. of turkey breast, boneless & skinless
- ¼ cup of vegetable oil
- 2 tbsp. of honey
- Half cup of lime juice
- 1 tsp of dried thyme
- 1 tsp of dried rosemary

Instructions

- In a bowl, mix all ingredients except for the turkey.
- Take out two tbsp. from marinade and set it aside
- Cut the turkey in half lengthwise so the pieces will be thinner.
- Add turkey in marinade, coat well, and chill in the fridge for 1 to 2 hours.
- Let the oven broiler preheat to 500 F
- Broil turkey on each side for four minutes.
- Baste turkey in 2 tbsp. of marinade while cooking.
- Serve hot.

Nutrient per serving: Calories: 245 g| Protein: 17.1 g| Carbohydrates: 11.5 g| Fiber: 0.4 g| Total Fat: 15 g| Sodium: 35 mg| Phosphorus: 131 mg| Potassium: 200 mg

5.28 Curried Turkey Casserole

Ingredients

- Broccoli florets: 3 cups
- Olive oil: 1/4 cup+ 2 tbsp.
- 2 cloves of minced garlic
- All-purpose flour: 1/4 cup
- One diced onion
- 2% milk: 1 cup
- Chicken broth, no salt: 2 cups
- Curry powder: 2 teaspoons
- 1 cup chopped bell peppers
- White bread: 3 cups, cut into cubes
- Black pepper
- Turkey: 4 cups, sliced into pieces

Instructions

- Let the oven preheat to 400 F
- In a pot, add oil sauté garlic, onion until tender for seven minutes.
- Add in flour and mix for one minute. Gradually add broth and milk, mixing continuously until it simmers.
- Add in black pepper, curry powder, peppers, broccoli cook for five minutes until softened. Add in cooked turkey.
- Place mixture in baking dish.

- In a bowl, add bread and oil, coat well. Add bread to the turkey mix.
- Bake for 15 minutes, until brown and bubbles.

Nutrient per Serving: Calories: 380 g| Protein: 26 g| Carbohydrates: 23 g| Fiber: 2 g| Total Fat: 20 g| Sodium: 113 mg| phosphorus: 227 mg| Potassium: 472 mg

5.29 Turkey Sliders with Peach Tarragon Aioli

Ingredients

- Ground turkey: 2 cups
- Parsley: 1/3 cup, chopped
- Garlic powder: 1 teaspoon
- Dijon mustard: half tablespoon
- Poultry seasoning: 1 teaspoon
- Half cup of arugula
- Six slider buns
- Red onion: 1/4 cup, diced

For Aioli

- Peaches: 2 tablespoons, pureed
- Low-fat mayonnaise: 2 tablespoons
- Tarragon: 1 teaspoon, chopped

Instructions

- Preheat grill on medium-high. In a bowl, add poultry season, red onion, mustard, turkey, garlic powder, parsley. Make it into six patties.

- Cook patties for 5 to 6 minutes on each side, until a meat thermometer, reads 165 F
- Meanwhile, make peach aioli mix all ingredients.
- Spread peach aioli on the slider, then patty and enjoy.

Nutrient per serving: Calories: 257 g| Protein: 16 g| Carbohydrates: 33 g| Fiber: 4 g| Total Fat: 11 g| sodium: 257 mg| Phosphorus: 240 mg| Potassium: 330 mg

5.30 Turkey Breast with Cranberry Orange Ginger Sauce

Ingredients

- Fresh parsley: 1 Tbsp.
- 4 lbs. of skin-on turkey breast
- Fresh thyme: 1 tsp
- Fresh rosemary: 1 tsp
- Salt: ¼ tsp
- Olive oil: ¼ cup
- Pepper: ¼ tsp
- Half tsp of lemon zest

Instructions

- Let the oven preheat to 350 F
- Mix herbs, oil, salt, and black pepper
- Loosen the turkey skin from flesh with your fingers.
- Place turkey in pan. Add 2 tbsp. Of oil mix under skin and secure with toothpicks.

- Pour the rest of the oil over the turkey breast.
- Cover it and roast for 1 to 1.5 hours.
- let the turkey rest for ten-15 minutes, pull the skin off, and discard

Nutrient per serving: Calories: 244.3 g| Protein: 32.6 g| Carbohydrates: 0.1 g| Fiber: 0.04 g| Total Fat: 11.8 g| Sodium: 108 mg| Phosphorus: 238 mg|

Potassium: 329 mg

5.31 Beef Schnitzel

Ingredients

- One lean beef schnitzel
- Olive oil: 2 tablespoon
- Breadcrumbs: ¼ cup
- One egg
- One lemon, to serve

Instructions

- Let the oven pre-heat to 400 F.
- In a big bowl, add breadcrumbs and oil, mix well until forms a crumbly mixture
- Dip beef steak in whisked egg and coat in breadcrumbs mixture.
- Place the breaded beef in the oven and cook for 20 minutes or more until fully cooked through.
- Take out from the oven and serve with the side of lemon.

Nutrition per serving: Calories 340 |Proteins 20g |Carbs 14g |Fat 10g |Fiber 7g

5.32 Mama's Meatloaf

Ingredients

- Ground lean beef: 4 cups
- Bread crumbs: 1 cup (soft and fresh)
- Chopped mushrooms: ½ cup
- Cloves of minced garlic
- Shredded carrots: ½ cup
- Beef broth: ¼ cup
- Chopped onions: ½ cup
- Two eggs beaten
- Ketchup: 3 Tbsp.
- Worcestershire sauce: 1 Tbsp.
- Dijon mustard: 1 Tbsp.

For Glaze

- Honey: ¼ cup
- Ketchup: half cup
- Dijon mustard: 2 tsp

Instructions

- In a big bowl, add beef broth and breadcrumbs, stir well. And set it aside in a food processor, add garlic, onions, mushrooms, and carrots, and pulse on high until finely chopped
- In a separate bowl, add soaked breadcrumbs, Dijon mustard, Worcestershire sauce, eggs, lean ground beef, ketchup, and salt.

- With your hands, combine well and make it into a loaf.
- Let the oven preheat to 390 F.
- Put Meatloaf in the oven and let it cook for 40 minutes.
- In the meantime, add Dijon mustard, ketchup, and brown sugar in a bowl and mix. Glaze this mix over Meatloaf when five minutes are left.
- Rest the Meatloaf after for ten minutes before serving.

Nutrition per serving: Calories 330 |Proteins 19g |Carbs 16g|Fat 9.9 g |

5.33 Steak with Broccoli Bundles

Ingredients

- Olive oil spray
- Flank steak (2 pounds)- cut into 6 pieces
- Kosher salt and black pepper
- Two cloves of minced garlic
- Broccoli florets: 2 and a half cups
- Tamari sauce: half cup
- Three bell peppers: sliced thinly
- Beef broth: 1/3 cup
- 1 Tbsp. of unsalted butter
- Balsamic vinegar: 1/4 cup

Instructions

- Sprinkle salt and pepper on steak and rub.

- In a zip lock bag, add garlic and Tamari sauce, then add steak, toss well and seal the bag.

- Let it marinate for one hour to overnight.

- Equally, place bell peppers and asparagus in the center of the steak.

- Roll the steak around the vegetables and secure well with toothpicks.

- Preheat the oven.

- Spray the steak with olive oil spray. And place steaks in the oven.

- Cook for 15 minutes at 400 F or more till steaks are cooked

- Take the steak out from the oven and let it rest for five minute

- Remove steak bundles and allow them to rest for 5 minutes before serving/slicing.

- In the meantime, add butter, balsamic vinegar, and broth over medium flame. Mix well and reduce it by half. Add salt and pepper to taste.

- Pour over steaks right before serving.

Nutrition per serving: Calories 471 |Proteins 29g |Carbs 20g |Fat 15g |

5.34 Beef Hamburger

Ingredients

- Buns:4

- Lean ground beef chuck: 4 cups

- Salt, to taste

- Slices of any cheese: 4 slices

- Black Pepper, to taste

Instructions

- Let the oven preheat to 350 F.

- In a bowl, add lean ground beef, pepper, and salt. Mix well and form patties.

- Put them in the oven in one layer only, cook for 6 minutes, flip them halfway through. One minute before you take out the patties add cheese on top.

- When cheese is melted, take out from the oven.

- Add ketchup, any dressing to your buns. Add tomatoes and lettuce and patties.

- Serve hot.

Nutrition per serving: Calories: 520kcal | Carbohydrates: 22g | Protein: 31g | Fat: 34g |

5.35 Beef Steak Kabobs with Vegetables

Ingredients

- Light sodium Soy sauce: 2 tbsp.

- Lean beef chuck ribs: 4 cups, cut into one-inch pieces

- Low-fat sour cream: 1/3 cup

- Half onion

- 8 skewers: 6 inch

- One bell peppers

Instructions

- In a mixing bowl, add soy sauce and sour cream, mix well. Add the lean beef chunks, coat well, and let it marinate for half an hour or more.

- Cut onion, bell pepper into one-inch pieces. In water, soak skewers for ten minutes.

- Add onions, bell peppers, and beef on skewers; alternatively, sprinkle with Black Pepper

- Let it cook for 10 minutes, in a preheated oven at 400F, flip halfway through.

- Serve with yogurt dipping sauce.

Nutrition per serving: Calories 268 |Proteins 20g |Carbs 15g|Fat 10g |

5.36 Beef Empanadas

Ingredients

- Square gyoza wrappers: eight pieces

- Olive oil: 1 tablespoon

- White onion: 1/4 cup, finely diced

- Mushrooms: 1/4 cup, finely diced

- Half cup lean ground beef

- Chopped garlic: 2 teaspoons

- Paprika: 1/4 teaspoon

- Ground cumin: 1/4 teaspoon

- Six green olives, diced

- Ground cinnamon: 1/8 teaspoon

- Diced tomatoes: half cup

- One egg, lightly beaten

Instructions

- In a skillet, over a medium flame, add oil, onions, and beef and cook for 3 minutes, until meat turns brown.

- Add mushrooms and cook for six minutes until it starts to brown. Then add paprika, cinnamon, olives, cumin, and garlic and cook for 3 minutes or more.

- Add in the chopped tomatoes and cook for a minute. Turn off the heat; let it cool for five minutes.

- Lay gyoza wrappers on a flat surface add one and a half tbsp. of beef filling in each wrapper. Brush edges with water or egg, fold wrappers, pinch edges.

- Put empanadas in the oven, and cook for 7 minutes at 400°F until nicely browned.

- Serve with sauce and salad greens.

Nutrition per serving: Calories 343 |Fat 19g |Protein 18g |Carbohydrate 12.9g

5.37 Rib-Eye Steak

Ingredients

- Lean rib eye steaks: 2, medium size

- Salt & freshly ground black pepper, to taste

Instructions

- Let the oven preheat at 400 F. pat dry steaks with paper towels.
- Use any spice blend or just salt and pepper on steaks.
- Generously on both sides of the steak.
- Put steaks in the oven. Cook according to the rareness you want. Or cook for 14 minutes and flip after half time.
- Take out from the oven and let it rest for about 5 minutes.
- Serve with salad.

Nutrition per serving: Calories: 470kcal | Protein: 45g | Fat: 31g | carbs: 23 g

5.38 Turkey Fajitas Platter

Ingredients

- Cooked Turkey Breast: 1/4 cup
- Six Tortilla Wraps
- One Yellow Pepper
- One Red Pepper
- Half Red Onion
- Soft Cheese: 5 Tbsp.
- Mexican Seasoning: 2 Tbsp.
- Cumin: 1 Tsp
- Kosher salt& Pepper
- Cajun Spice: 3 Tbsp.
- Fresh Coriander

Instructions

- Slice the vegetables.
- Dice up turkey breast into small bite-size pieces.
- In a bowl, add onions, turkey, soft cheese, and peppers along with seasonings. Mix it well.
- Place it in foil and the oven.
- Cook for 20 minutes at 200C.
- Serve hot.

Nutrition per serving: Calories: 379kcal | Carbohydrates: 84g | Protein: 30g | Fat: 39g |

5.39 Turkey Breast Tenderloin

Ingredients

- Turkey breast tenderloin: one-piece
- Thyme: half tsp.
- Sage: half tsp.
- Paprika: half tsp.
- Pink salt: half tsp.
- Freshly ground black pepper: half tsp.

Instructions

- Let the oven preheat to 350 F
- In a bowl, mix all the spices and herbs, rub it all over the turkey.
- Put the turkey in the oven and let it cook at 350 F for 25 minutes, flip halfway through.
- Serve with salad.

5.40 Turkey Breast with Maple Mustard Glaze

Ingredients

- Whole turkey breast: 5 pounds
- Olive oil: 2 tsp.
- Maple syrup: 1/4 cup
- Dried sage: half tsp.
- Smoked paprika: half tsp.
- Dried thyme: one tsp.
- Salt: one tsp.
- Freshly ground black pepper: half tsp.
- Dijon mustard: 2 tbsp.

Instructions

- Let the oven preheat to 350 F
- Rub the olive oil all over the turkey breast
- In a bowl, mix salt, sage, pepper, thyme, and paprika. Mix well and coat turkey in this spice rub.
- Place the turkey in an oven, cook for 25 minutes at 350°F. Flip the turkey over and cook for another 12 minutes. Flip again and cook for another ten minutes. With an instant-read thermometer, the internal temperature should reach 165°F.
- In the meantime, in a saucepan, mix mustard, maple syrup, and with one tsp. of butter.
- Brush this glaze all over the turkey when cooked.
- Cook again for five minutes. Slice and Serve with salad green.

Nutrition per serving: Cal 379 | Fat: 23 g| Carbs: 21g | Protein: 52g

5.41 Juicy Turkey Burgers with Zucchini

Ingredients

- Gluten-free breadcrumbs: 1/4 cup(seasoned)
- Grated zucchini: 1 cup
- Red onion: 1 tbsp. (grated)
- Lean ground turkey: 4 cups
- One clove of minced garlic
- 1 tsp of kosher salt and fresh pepper

Instructions

- In a bowl, add zucchini (moisture removed with a paper towel), ground turkey, garlic, salt, onion, pepper, breadcrumbs. Mix well
- With your hands, makes five patties. But not too thick.
- Let the oven preheat to 375 F
- Put in an oven in a single layer and cook for 7 minutes or more. Until cooked through and browned.

- Place in buns with ketchup and lettuce and enjoy.

Nutrition per serving: Calories: 161kcal|Carbohydrates: 4.5g| Protein: 18g|Fat: 7g|

5.42 Oven Turkey Breast

Ingredients

- Turkey breast: 4 pounds, ribs removed, bone with skin
- Olive oil: 1 tablespoon
- Salt: 2 teaspoons
- Dry turkey seasoning (without salt): half tsp.

Instructions

- Rub half tbsp. Of olive oil over turkey breast. Sprinkle salt, turkey seasoning on both sides of turkey breast with half tbsp. of olive oil.
- Let the oven preheat at 350 F. put turkey skin side down in the oven and cook for 20 minutes until the turkey's temperature reaches 160 F for half an hour to 40 minutes.
- Let it sit for ten minutes before slicing.
- Serve.

Nutrition per serving: Calories: 226kcal| Protein: 32.5g|Fat: 10g|carbs 22 g

5.43 Turkey & Noodles

Ingredients

- Dry elbow macaroni: 2 cups

- Olive oil: 1 tablespoon
- 2 pounds of lean ground turkey
- Half cup of diced green onions
- Half cup of chopped green pepper
- Italian seasoning: 1 tablespoon
- Black pepper: 1 teaspoon
- Canned tomatoes, no salt: one cup

Instructions

- Cook pasta as per instructions.
- In a pan, brown the turkey in heated olive oil.
- Add bell peppers, tomatoes, seasoning, black pepper, cooked macaroni, and onions. Mix well.
- Cover and let it simmer for five minutes. Serve right away

Nutrition per serving: 273 calories | 188 mg sodium|33 g protein| 80 mg cholesterol| 533 mg potassium|7 g total fat |22 g carbohydrates |296 mg phosphorus| 1 g saturated fat |2 g fiber| 55 mg calcium

5.44 Rotini with Mock Italian Sausage

Ingredients

- ¾ Pound of lean ground turkey
- Half cup uncooked rotini pasta
- ¾ teaspoon of Italian seasoning
- 1 cup diced onion
- Half cup of celery, chopped

- 1 clove of minced garlic
- One cup of red bell pepper, chopped
- Crushed red pepper: ¼ teaspoon
- Tomato paste, no salt added: 3 tablespoons
- Grated parmesan cheese: 2 tablespoons
- Fennel seeds: ¼ teaspoon

Instructions

- Cook pasta as per instructions. Set it aside
- Cook turkey until browned. Drain with paper towels.
- Add celery, seasonings, and onion—Cook for three minutes.
- Add tomato paste, bell pepper. Lower the heat, partially cover, and simmer for 15 minutes.
- Serve over pasta.

Nutrition per serving: 165 calories | 250 mg sodium| 13 g protein| 41 mg cholesterol |458 mg potassium| 2 g total fat| 28 g carbohydrate |161 mg phosphorus| 1 gram saturated fat |2 g fiber| 65 mg calcium

5.45 Turkey New Orleans style

Ingredients

- Vegetable oil: 2 tablespoons
- Green peppers: ¼ cup diced
- 1-pound lean ground turkey
- Half tsp. Of cayenne pepper

- All-purpose flour: 2 tablespoons
- 1 clove of minced garlic
- Celery: ¼ cup, chopped
- Onion: ¼ cup diced
- Cooked rice: 2 cups
- Green onions: ¼ cup diced
- Chicken broth, low sodium: 1 cup

Instructions

- Let the oven preheat to 350 F
- Cook meat until browned in hot oil. Drain on a paper towel.
- Add flour and stir until light brown. Add peppers, onions, garlic, and celery. Cook till vegetables are soft.
- Add meat, rice to the pan.
- Add a little broth, so it's not too wet.
- Add into the baking dish.
- Bake for 18-20 minutes.

Nutrition per serving: 393 calories | 113 mg sodium|27 g protein| 84 mg cholesterol |377 mg potassium|19 g total fat |28 g carbohydrate| 228 mg phosphorus|4 g saturated| 1 g fiber |43 mg calcium

5.46 Barbecue Cups

Ingredients

- One package of low-fat biscuits
- Lean ground turkey: ¾ pounds
- Onion flakes: 2 teaspoons

- Half cup of spicy barbecue sauce
- Dash of garlic powder

Instructions

- In a skillet, brown the meat.
- Add garlic powder, barbecue sauce, and onion flakes, mix it well
- Add biscuits and press in the muffin tin
- Add meat mixture in the center.
- Bake for 10-12 minutes, at 400°F.

Nutrition per serving: 134 calories | 342 mg sodium|7 g protein| 27 mg cholesterol |151 mg potassium|5 g total fat |13 g carbohydrate| 152 mg phosphorus|1 g saturated fat| 0 g fiber| 11 mg calcium

5.47 Low Sodium Beef Stew Recipe

Ingredients

- 2 diced celery stalks
- 2 to 3 lbs. of stew meat, cut in one-inch pieces, boneless
- One diced onion
- One carrot sliced
- 2 cloves of minced garlic
- Tomato paste, no salt added: 3 tablespoons
- Frozen peas: 1 cup
- Red cooking wine: 1 cup
- One bay leaf
- Dijon mustard: 2 tablespoons, low sodium
- Beef broth, low sodium: 1 and a half cups
- Black pepper: 1 teaspoon
- Fresh parsley: 2 tablespoons, chopped
- Dried thyme: 1 teaspoon

Instructions

- Add oil to a large frying pan and bring to a simmer over medium heat. Add celery, carrots, onion, garlic, and thyme, occasionally stirring for about 10 minutes until the carrots just begin to soften.
- Add tomato paste, mustard, and wine, and stir well. Simmer for 5-10 minutes until the wine reduces by about half. Remove from heat and set aside.
- In a slow cooker, add meat, beef broth, pepper, and wine/vegetable mixture. Make sure meat is coated.
- Stir in the bay leaf, cover, and cook on high for 5-6 hours. Stir every hour, if possible.
- Add frozen peas and fresh parsley at the very end, about 10 minutes before serving.

Nutrients per serving: calories 124| total fat 1.8 g| saturated fat 0.0 g| monounsaturated fat 0.5 g| cholesterol 38 mg| calcium 7.8 mg| sodium 32 mg|

phosphorus 89 mg| potassium 78 mg| | protein 12.9 g

5.48 Roast Turkey with Fresh Sage

- Olive oil: 1 teaspoon
- One fresh turkey of 12 pound
- Half diced yellow onion
- One bunch of fresh sage
- Poultry seasoning: 2 teaspoons

Instructions

- Remove turkey neck, giblets from the turkey cavity. Wash and pat dry.
- Add poultry seasoning in the cavity, add sage and onion.
- Grease the roasting pan and place turkey.
- Let the oven preheat to 350 F, bake for 2.5-3 hours, cook until juices run clear.
- Take out from the oven, cover with aluminum foil,
- Let it rest for 20 minutes, then serve.

Nutrients per serving: calories 134| total fat 2.8 g| saturated fat 0.9 g| monounsaturated fat 0.5 g| polyunsaturated fat 0.7 g| cholesterol 59 mg| calcium 16 mg| sodium 54 mg| phosphorus 186 mg| potassium 259 mg| | protein 25 g

5.49 Broccoli & Beef Stir-Fry

Ingredients

- Cooked rice: 2 cups
- 2 cloves of garlic, minced
- One cup of uncooked lean sirloin beef, cut into strips
- Olive oil: 2 tablespoons
- One and a half cups of frozen broccoli
- One small roma tomato, chopped
- Chicken broth, low-sodium: 1/4 cup
- Soy sauce, reduced-sodium: 2 tablespoons
- Cornstarch: 1 tablespoon

Instructions

- Thaw the broccoli.
- In a pan, sauté garlic for one minute, add broccoli, cook for five minutes. Take out from the pan and set it aside.
- In the same pan, add meat, cook to your desired likeness.
- In a bowl, mix soy sauce, chicken broth, and cornstarch.
- Add vegetables, tomato, and sauce to the beef. Cook and stir until sauce is thick.
- Serve with a half cup of rice.

Nutrients per serving: Calories 373| Protein 18 g| Carbohydrates 37 g| Fat 17 g| Cholesterol 42 mg| Sodium 351 mg| Potassium 555 mg| Phosphorus 255 mg| Calcium 62 mg| Fiber 5.1 g

5.50 Italian Beef with Peppers & Onions

Ingredients

- 1 tsp. of garlic powder
- Lean beef roast: 3-pound, fat trimmed
- 1 tsp. of crushed red pepper
- Black pepper: 2 teaspoons
- One sliced onion
- Oregano: 2 teaspoons
- Half cup of pepperoncini juice
- One diced green bell pepper, one red, one yellow

Instructions

- In a crockpot, add black pepper, red pepper, beef roast, garlic powder, oregano. Cook for 4-5 hours on high until soft enough.
- Take out from the pot, shred the meat, and remove the fat.
- Add shredded beef to the pot again, add onions, pepperoncini juice, and peppers.
- Cook for 50-60 minutes, on high, until vegetables are tender.

Nutrients per serving: Calories 212| Protein 25 g| Carbohydrates 3 g| Fat 11 g| Cholesterol 84 mg| Sodium 121 mg| Potassium 280 mg| Phosphorus 196 mg| Calcium 21 mg| Fiber 0.6 g

5.51 Braised Beef Brisket

Ingredients

- Beef broth, reduced-sodium: 2 cups
- Half medium onion, chopped
- One carrot, chopped
- Fresh parsley: 1 tablespoon, chopped
- Two and a half pounds of beef brisket (trimmed fat)
- One stalk of celery, chopped
- Black pepper: 2 teaspoons
- 3 bay leaves. Crumbled
- 3 cups of water
- Two tablespoons of balsamic vinegar
- Canola oil: 2 tablespoons

Instructions

- Let the oven preheat to 350° F.
- Sprinkle the beef with black pepper.
- In a Dutch oven, brown beef for five minutes on every side in hot oil over medium heat.
- Take out the meat and add carrots, onion, and celery.
- Cook for four minutes.
- Add parsley and bay leaves to the vegetable mix, and put meat on top of the vegetables.
- Add water, broth, and balsamic vinegar.
- Let it boil.

- Cover the pot and cook in the oven for one and a half hours. Flip the meat over and cook a one and a half hours more until beef is soft enough to shred with a fork.

- Take the meat out from the pot. Store broth for gravy

- Serve the brisket.

Nutrients per serving: Calories 230| Protein 29 g| Carbohydrates 4 g| Fat 11 g| Cholesterol 84 mg| Sodium 178 mg| Potassium 346 mg| Phosphorus 193 mg| Calcium 30 mg| Fiber 0.8 g|

Chapter 6: Kidney-Friendly Fish & Seafood Recipes

6.1 Tuna Fish Salad with Fennel & Orange Salsa

Ingredients

- Garlic-infused olive oil: 2 teaspoons
- Smoked paprika: 1 teaspoon
- Ground coriander: 1 teaspoon
- Salt: ¼ teaspoon
- Black pepper: 1/8 teaspoon
- Fresh tuna steak: 5 cups
- olive oil: 1 teaspoon
- Fennel bulb (1 bulb)
- Olive oil: 3 tablespoons
- Two oranges
- Five olives: chopped
- Parsley: 2 tablespoons
- Dried oregano: ½ teaspoon
- Cider vinegar: 2 tablespoons
- Thinly sliced scallion greens: ¼ cup
- Salt: 1/16 teaspoon
- Black pepper

Instructions

- Combine the smoked paprika, two tsp. Of garlic-infused oil, salt, coriander, and pepper into a shallow dish. Brush the tuna steak with the spice mixture on both sides and put aside.

- Break off fennel bulb stalks and throw them away. Slice pieces of fennel into 1/4 inch of the neck and put them in one layer on the baking sheet. Drizzle with two teaspoons of oil.

- Roast for about 11 to 13 minutes, till the fennel becomes medium golden brown. turn the pieces over and brown for five minutes, take out from the oven and cool it down

- Zest the orange it into a serving bowl, add 1/4 cup of orange juice. chop up another orange

- Add the oregano, juice, olives, sliced orange bits, parsley, cider vinegar, salt and peppers, scallions, two tablespoons remaining of garlic-infused liquid the orange zest.

- Coarsely chop and whisk the cooked, roasted fennel into the orange salsa.

- Preheat medium-heat a large skillet; drizzle with canola oil.

- Add the tuna steaks to the skillet and cook for five minutes until browned at the rim. Switch on the other side and cook for four minutes.

- Take the tuna off from the heat Break the tuna into pieces, following 2 or 3 minutes of rest.

- Cover 1/2 cup of Roasted Fennel Orange Salsa, then finish with 1/4 of the seared tuna strips.

Nutrition Per Serving: 351 calories| total fat 16 g | carbohydrates 14.4 g| protein 23 g | Cholesterol 4.1 mg| Sodium 142 mg| potassium 132 mg| Phosphorus 121 mg |Calcium 45 mg| Fiber 2.1 g

6.2 Baked Fish with Roasted Sweet Potatoes & Mushroom

Ingredients

- Wild Salmon: 1 and ½ cup, cut into four pieces
- sweet potatoes cubed: 2 cups, leached
- Olive oil divided: two tbsp.
- Salt: ¼ tsp.
- Herbs: 1 tsp.
- Mushrooms: 4 cups(sliced)
- Two cloves garlic: sliced
- Lemon juice: 4 tbsp.
- Ground pepper: ¼ tsp.
- Thyme

Instructions

- Let the oven heat till 425 F
- Add one tbsp. Of oil, potatoes, mushroom, pepper, and salt in a bowl.
- Transfer it to a baking dish and roast for almost forty minutes until the vegetables are soft. Stir the vegetables and add. garlic

- Place fish over it. Drizzle with one tbsp. Of oil, lemon juice. Sprinkle with herbs bake till fish is flaky for fifteen minutes.

Nutrition Per Serving: 275 calories| total fat 16.8 g | carbohydrates 15.4 g| protein 21.3 g | Cholesterol 5.3 mg| Sodium 132 mg| potassium 141 mg| Phosphorus 111 mg |Calcium 56 mg| Fiber 2.3 g

6.3 Swordfish with Olives, Capers over Polenta

Ingredients

- Chopped red peppers: 2 Cups
- Half cup of regular or coarse yellow cornmeal
- Swordfish: 4 cups, cut into four steaks
- 2 and ½ cups of water
- Extra-virgin olive oil: 1 tablespoon
- Chopped fresh basil: 3 tablespoons
- 4 medium stalks celery, chopped
- ¼ of cup green olives pitted and roughly diced
- Capers: 1 tablespoon rinsed
- A pinch of crushed red pepper
- Half teaspoon of salt, divided
- 2 cloves of pressed garlic
- For garnish Fresh basil
- Freshly ground black pepper: ⅛ teaspoon

Instructions

- Put a saucepan over medium flame and boil two cups of water with 1/4 tsp. of salt. Add the cornmeal carefully to avoid any lumps.

- Cook for three minutes, keep stirring.

- Lower the heat. Stir after every five minutes, cook for 20-25 minutes. If it becomes too hard, add a half cup of water, turn off the heat but keep it covered.

- In the meantime, in a large skillet over a medium flame, add in the oil. Add celery fry it, frequently stirring, until soft, for around five minutes.

- Then add garlic, cook for almost 30 seconds. Add in olives, bell peppers, basil, crushed red pepper, capers, freshly ground black pepper and the remaining 1/4 tsp. of Sea salt.

- Cover it lower the heat and cook for five minutes.

- Add swordfish in the sauce. Let it simmer, and Cover it cook for 10-15 minutes, till swordfish is cooked completely.

- On a serving tray, layer the cornmeal at the bottom. Add the fish over the cornmeal, cover with the sauce and, garnish with fresh basil, serve hot and enjoy

Nutrition Per Serving: 276 calories| total fat 12.1 g | carbohydrates 13.2 g| protein 22 g | Cholesterol 5.3 mg| Sodium 131 mg| potassium 124 mg| Phosphorus 104 mg |Calcium 46 mg| Fiber 2.4 g

6.4 Salmon Souvlaki Bowls

Ingredients

- 4 cups of fresh salmon sliced into four pieces

- Fresh oregano: 1 tablespoon

- Lemon juice: 6 tablespoons

- vinegar: 2 tablespoons

- Smoked paprika: 1 tablespoon or regular paprika

- Fresh dill: 1 tablespoon

- Three tablespoons of extra virgin olive oil

- 2 cloves of minced garlic minced

- Half teaspoon of salt

- One teaspoon of black pepper

- Two cucumbers cut in sliced

- Dry pearl couscous: 1 cup

- Half cup of Kalamata olives

- One-inch zucchini cut into 1/4 rounds

- Juice from one lemon

- Extra virgin olive oil: 2 tablespoons

- Red peppers: 2 pieces, quartered

Instructions

- Mix balsamic vinegar, oregano, smoked paprika, black pepper, garlic, salt, olive oil, dill, and lemon juice in a big mixing bowl and mix until well combined

- Pour this marinade all over the salmon, rub gently and make sure the salmon is covered in marinade. Let it rest for 15 minutes.

- In the meantime, cook couscous to your liking.

- Mix two tablespoons of olive oil, red peppers, black pepper, salt, and zucchini in a mixing bowl. Mix well to coat the vegetables.

- Let the grill/grill pan heat up over medium flame.

- Grill the salmon on each side for about three minutes. Or cook to your liking.

- After salmon, grill zucchini, bell peppers for four minutes each side so the grill marks will appear.

- Take serving bowls, add faro or couscous on the bottom, add lemon juice to coat couscous. Then add salmon, olives, grilled veggies, cucumbers.

- Add any of your favorite sauce or Tzatziki sauce, add fresh herbs and serve.

Nutrition Per Serving: 244 calories| total fat 14 g | carbohydrates 17.1g| protein 21 g | Cholesterol 6.1 mg| So-
dium 131 mg| potassium 120 mg| Phosphorus 109 mg |Calcium 48.2 mg| Fiber 2.2 g

6.5 Mediterranean Tuna- Salad

Ingredients

- One can of 5 ounces, drained chunk light tuna in water

- One and ½ tablespoons of water

- 4 Kalamata olives, pitted, diced

- Feta cheese crumbled: 2 tablespoons

- One and ½ tablespoons of tahini

- One and ½ tablespoons of lemon juice

- Parsley: 2 tablespoons

- One medium orange, sliced(peeled)

Instructions

- In a bowl, whisk together the water, tahini, and lemon juice. Add salmon, olives, parsley, and feta, toss to combine.

- Serve right away the tuna salad with the orange wedges on the side, with a cup of kale.

Nutrition Per Serving: 275 calories| total fat 11.4 g | carbohydrates 13.2 g| protein 21 g | Cholesterol 5.3 mg| Sodium 134 mg| potassium 142 mg| Phosphorus 119.9 mg |Calcium 52 mg| Fiber 2.9 g

6.6 Salmon Bowl with Faro, Green Beans, & Tahini Dressing

Ingredients

- Extra-virgin olive oil: 6 tablespoons divided
- Half of a cup cooked green beans
- Salmon: 3/4 cup
- Tahini: 2 tablespoons
- Zest and juice of one lemon
- ¼ of teaspoon garlic powder
- Half teaspoon of turmeric, divided
- Faro: ¼ cup
- Half of teaspoon cumin
- One and ½ teaspoons smoked paprika
- 2 scallions, thinly chopped
- Half teaspoon of coriander
- 4 pieces' lettuce leaves
- Fresno Chile: ¼ of a whole, thinly sliced
- Kosher salt and freshly ground black pepper

Instructions

- Mix lemon zest, the tahini, lemon juice, garlic powder, and ¼ teaspoon of Turmeric and a big bowl.
- Slowly add three tablespoons of olive oil and mix until smooth and fully emulsified for the sauce. Adjust salt and pepper.
- Put a small pot over medium flame, add the faro, and one cup of water. Let it boil. Lower the heat and let it simmer for 20 -25 minutes until the faro is soft. Set it aside.
- In a bowl, add one tablespoon of olive oil, the beans, and the cumin mix well set it aside.
- With smoked paprika, ¼ teaspoon of turmeric, coriander, salt, and pepper mix it and season the salmon with this pace mix.
- Heat the remaining two tablespoons of olive oil over a low flame in a medium skillet. Add in the salmon and cook for about five minutes until lightly browned on one side and opaque in the middle.
- Lay lettuce leaves at the bottom of a serving bowl. Add Faro, salmon, and green beans. Garnish with the slices of the scallions, and the diced chili add dressing on top

Nutrition Per Serving: 351 calories| total fat 18.2 g | carbohydrates 12.3 g| protein 17.1 g | Cholesterol 5.1 mg| Sodium 141 mg| potassium 113 mg| Phosphorus 109 mg |Calcium 47.2 mg| Fiber 2.4 g

6.7 Salmon Pita Sandwich

Ingredients

- Pita bread: half (6 inches)
- Chopped fresh dill: 2 teaspoons
- Half of a teaspoon prepared horseradish
- Nonfat yogurt: 2 tablespoons(plain)
- Flaked canned sockeye salmon: 6 tbsp.(drained)
- Half of a cup watercress
- Lemon juice: 2 teaspoons

Instructions

- In a small mixing bowl, mix lemon juice, yogurt, horseradish, and dill.
- Mix well.
- Add in the salmon.
- Put the salmon salad into a pita pocket with watercress.
- Serve right away, enjoy.

Nutrition Per Serving: 239 calories| total fat 7.1 g | carbohydrates 12.3 g| protein 19.4 g | Cholesterol 5.1 mg| Sodium 132 mg| potassium 138 mg| Phosphorus 131 mg |Calcium 52 mg| Fiber 3 g

6.8 Smoked Salmon & Poached Eggs on Toast

Ingredients

With sesame seeds & soy sauce

- Lemon juice: 1/4 tsp
- Salt & pepper to taste
- Smoked salmon: 3.5 oz.
- Scallions: 1 TBSP (sliced)
- Bread toasted: 2 slices
- Two poached eggs
- Dash of soy sauce
- Microgreens is optional

Everything bagel seasoning with tomato

- Avocado: 1/2
- Bread: 2 slices
- Lemon juice: 1/4 tsp
- Smoked salmon: 3.5 oz.
- Two poached eggs
- Salt & pepper to taste
- Two thin slices of tomatoes
- Microgreens are also optional.
- Everything Bagel Seasoning: 1 tsp

Instructions

- Smash the Avocado in a dish. Add a pinch of salt and lemon juice; combine properly, and put aside.
- Poach your eggs, and toast your bread as the eggs rest in the ice water
- Place the Avocado on both slices once your bread is toasted, then add the smoked salmon to each piece.
- Place the poached eggs gently on each of the toast.

- Add a drop of Kikkoman soy sauce and some crushed pepper, scallion, and microgreen garnish.

Nutrition Per Serving: 201 calories| total fat 12.3 g | carbohydrates 6.9 g| protein 12.7 g | Cholesterol 3.1 mg| Sodium 141 mg| potassium 126 mg| Phosphorus 112 mg |Calcium 47 mg| Fiber 2.8 g

6.9 Mediterranean Couscous with Tuna & Pepperoncini

Ingredients

For Couscous

- One and ¼ cups couscous
- One cup of chicken broth or water
- ¾ teaspoon of kosher salt

For Accompaniments

- ¼ of a cup capers
- Two cans oil-packed tuna: 5-ounce each
- Half of a cup sliced pepperoncini
- ⅓ of a cup chopped fresh parsley
- Extra-virgin olive oil, for serving
- One lemon wedges
- Kosher salt and freshly ground black pepper

Instructions

- To Make the Couscous: Put a small saucepan over medium heat, add broth or water to the pan let it boil. Turn off the heat, add the couscous, and let it rest for ten minutes.
- To make the accompaniments: In the meantime, add the tuna, pepperoncini, capers, and parsley in a small bowl and mix.
- With the help of a fork, fluff the couscous, sprinkle pepper, salt, and olive oil in it, and mix well.
- On a serving plate, put couscous on the bottom, add the tuna mix on top, drizzle lemon juice and serve with lemon slices.

Nutrition Per Serving: 226 calories| total fat 4g | carbohydrates 12.3 g| protein 8.4 g | Cholesterol 4.1 mg| Sodium 131 mg| potassium 133 mg| Phosphorus 112 mg |Calcium 43 mg| Fiber 2.6 g

6.10 Salmon Cakes

Ingredients

- One tablespoon of oil
- Garlic (minced): 1/2 tsp
- Salmon: 5 oz. cooked and finely diced
- Smoked paprika: 1/4 tsp
- 3 - 4 tablespoon of flour
- Fine kosher or sea salt: 1/4 tsp
- Curry powder: 1/4 tsp (optional)
- One sprig of rosemary

- Black pepper: 1/4 tsp
- Two egg whites

Instructions

- Mashup the salmon. remove any skin, if any
- Put the salmon in a bowl, then add the mashed veggies.
- Then add one tbsp. at a time in flour. Depending on the kind of salmon you choose, you'll need just 3-4 tbsp. Then add in herbs and seasonings. Mix well.
- Finally, add in two eggs.
- Mix well that the batter gets thick enough for patties to shape. Add one tbsp. More flour if the batter is too liquid.
- Shape into small or larger balls. then turn them into patties
- Turn the skillet on to medium flame add butter
- When hot, put in at least three or four cakes at a time. Cook on either side for almost four minutes, or until the salmon is fully cooked. Canned salmon cooks early, repeat the frying process for the rest of the cakes.
- Garnish with black pepper, rosemary, chili flakes, and a sprinkle of garlic if needed, serve hot.

Nutrition Per Serving: 91 calories| total fat 4 g | carbohydrates 6 g| protein 10 g | Cholesterol 4.3 mg| Sodium 101 mg| potassium 89 mg| Phosphorus 87 mg |Calcium 33 mg| Fiber 2.8 g

6.11 Salmon Parcels with Wild Rice, Pesto, & Broccoli

Ingredients

- Salmon fillets: one cup
- rice: one cup
- Red pesto: 3 tablespoon
- One lemon: half juiced and half thinly sliced
- Purple sprouting broccoli: half cup
- Black olives chopped: 2 tablespoon
- Basil

Instructions

- Let the overheat till 200 C to gas6, a 180 C. line the baking tray with parchment paper. Separate the mixed grains and rice. Stir in the lemon juice, olives, 2 tbsp. of pesto, and half of the basil. Mix well, put in the center of the baking tray
- Place the salmon over the grains and scatter over each fillet the remaining pesto. Cover with the slices of lemon and broccoli, then cover with parchment paper on top. make it a packet around filling
- Roast for about half an hour in the oven till broccoli is soft and salmon is completely cooked
- Serve with basil on top.

Nutrition Per Serving: 361 calories| total fat 16.2 g | carbohydrates 18 g| protein 9 g | Cholesterol 5.1 mg| Sodium 114 mg| potassium 121 mg| Phosphorus 109 mg |Calcium 56 mg| Fiber 3.2 g

6.12 Fish Taco Bowls with Chipotle Aioli over Cauliflower Rice

Ingredients

Blackened Fish

- Olive oil: 1 tablespoon
- Tilapia loins: 2 piece
- Salt: ½ tsp
- Smoked paprika: 1/2 tsp.
- Onion powder: 1/2 tsp.
- Chili powder: 1 tsp.
- Cumin: ¼ tsp
- Pepper: 1/4 teaspoon
- Garlic powder: 1/2 tsp.

Chipotle aioli

- Adobo sauce: 1 teaspoon
- Garlic powder: 1/2 tsp.
- Lime juice: ¼ tsp
- Low fat Mayonnaise: 1/4 tbsp.
- Chipotle pepper (in adoboe sauce): 1 tsp
- Soy milk: 1 tablespoon (full-fat)
- Salt: 1 tsp

Red Cabbage Slaw

- Half piece of a lime juiced

- Head red cabbage: 2 cups, sliced
- Salt: 1 tsp

Instructions

For Fish

- In a shallow bowl, mix all the spices and brush gently over the top and bottom of fish fillets.
- Heat the skillet over a medium flame, add coconut oil, then add fish.
- Look on either side for around four minutes, or until the fish flakes. don't let the fish overcook

Chipotle (Aioli)

- In a food processor, mix all the ingredients and pulse until creamy. Taste and mix with more salt or lime juice. if needed

Red Cabbage Slaw

- Mix all ingredients in a small bowl. mix lime juice and salt onto cabbage with your hands to tenderize before purple juices start oozing out
- Assemble your Fish Taco Bowls:
- Put coconut-lime Cauliflower rice in a bowl. Add red cabbage slaw with cauliflower rice. Cover with fish fillet, mango salsa, guacamole. while serving, add chipotle sauce.

Nutrition Per Serving: 239 calories| total fat 11 g | carbohydrates 21 g| protein 17 g | Cholesterol 5.6 mg| Sodium 121 mg| potassium 105 mg| Phosphorus 110 mg |Calcium 51 mg| Fiber 3.1 g

6.13 Fish Fajita

Ingredients

- 1 and 1/2 tsp. olive oil
- Fish: 4 cups
- One yellow, one red, one orange sliced bell peppers
- One tsp. of kosher salt
- Garlic powder: 1/2 tsp.
- Chili powder: 2 teaspoon
- Ground cumin: 1/2 teaspoon
- Lime
- Black pepper
- Cilantro
- Smoked paprika: 1/2 tsp
- Tortillas
- Onion powder: 1/2 teaspoon
- One onion sliced

Instructions

- Let the oven pre-heat to 450 F
- Add the fish, onion, olive oil, bell pepper, pepper, and salt, spices into a big bowl. mix well
- Spray oil on a baking sheet
- On that baking sheet, arrange the bell peppers, shrimp, and onions.

- Cook for about eight minutes, at 450 F. Switch the oven to broil, cook for another two minutes or until fish is completely cooked
- Squeeze lime juice over it and finish with coriander.
- Put in a warm tortilla and serve.

Nutrition Per Serving: 184 calories| total fat 9 g | carbohydrates 21 g| protein 13 g | Cholesterol 7.1 mg| Sodium 114 mg| potassium 123 mg| Phosphorus 104 mg |Calcium 45 mg| Fiber 2.8 g

6.14 Salmon with Green Bean Pilaf

Ingredients

- Olive oil: 3 tbsp.
- Pre-cooked white rice: one cup
- Wild salmon: 1 & ¼ pound (skinned and cut into four pieces)
- Green beans and cut into thirds: 12 ounces
- Low fat Mayonnaise: 2 tbsp.
- Minced garlic: one tbsp.
- Pine nuts: 2 tbsp.
- Water: 2 tbsp.
- Salt: ¾ tsp.
- Ground pepper: half tsp.
- Parsley
- Whole-grain mustard: 2 tsp.
- One lemon: zested, cut into wedges

Instructions

- Let the oven pre-heat till 425 F.
- Place parchment paper on baking sheet
- Brush the salmon with one spoonful of oil and place them on the baking sheet.
- Mash the salt and garlic together. In a small bowl, combine one teaspoon of the garlic paste with mustard, mayonnaise, 1/4 teaspoon of pepper.
- Spread the blend over the fish.
- Roast the salmon until it flakes easily — six-eight minutes per inch of thickness.
- Heat the remaining two spoons of oil over medium flame in a skillet.
- Add lemon zest, green beans, pine nuts, leftover garlic paste, and black pepper; stir for almost four minutes until the beans are soft.
- Reduce to medium heat. Add the rice and water and cook for three minutes, stirring, until hot.
- Serve with green beans and lemon and top with parsley.

Nutrition Per Serving: 242 calories| total fat 17.1 g | carbohydrates 18.1 g| protein 21.1 g | Cholesterol 6.1 mg| Sodium 125 mg| potassium 113 mg| Phosphorus 127 mg |Calcium 56 mg| Fiber 2.1 g

6.15 Fish Tacos with Broccoli Slaw & Cumin Sour Cream

Ingredients

- Eight tortillas
- Fish sticks: 2 10-oz. Packages
- Half red onion sliced
- Two limes, juiced and wedges
- Broccoli: 12 ounces
- Kosher salt: 1 tsp.
- Olive oil: 2 tablespoons
- Half cup of sour cream
- Cilantro: 1 cup
- Half tsp. of ground cumin

Instructions

- According to the direction on the package, cook the fish sticks.
- Chop broccoli' heads. Peel the stalks and cut them into matchsticks.
- In a large bowl, add the lime juice, onion, and 3⁄4 teaspoon of salt., mix and set aside around ten minutes.
- Add broccoli stalks and tops, oil, cilantro, and mix
- Mix cumin, sour cream, and salt in a small dish. Serve with fish

Nutrition Per Serving: 227 calories| total fat 14 g | carbohydrates 12.5 g| protein 20.3 g | Cholesterol 7.1 mg| Sodium 120 mg| potassium 109 mg| Phosphorus 102 mg |Calcium 6.1 mg| Fiber 3 g

6.16 Roasted Salmon with Smoky Chickpeas & Greens

Ingredients

- Wild salmon: 1 and ¼ pounds, cut in 4 pieces
- Chopped kale: 10 cups
- Olive oil: 2 tbsp.
- Salt: half tsp.
- Can of chickpeas: 15 ounces
- Garlic powder: ¼ tsp.
- Buttermilk: 1/3 cup
- Low fat Mayonnaise: ¼ cup
- Smoked paprika: one tbsp.
- Water: ¼ cup
- Ground pepper: half tsp.
- Chives: ¼ cup

Instructions

- let the oven pre-heat 'til 425 F and put the racks in the upper third portion, middle of the oven
- In a bowl, add one spoon of paprika, oil, 1/4 tsp of salt.
- Dry the chickpeas and mix with the paprika blend, put them on a baking sheet, and bake for half an hour on the upper rack.
- In the food, blender adds puree buttermilk, basil, mayonnaise,1/4 tsp of pepper, and garlic powder pulse till creamy. Set it aside.
- Heat a skillet, add one tablespoon of oil over medium flame.
- Add the kale, cook for two minutes. Add water and keep cooking, around five minutes until the kale is soft.
- Remove from flame, and add salt in the dish.
- Take out the chickpeas from the oven, transfer them to one side of the pan. Place the salmon on the other hand, and season with salt and pepper.
- Bake for 5- 8 minutes until the salmon is completely cooked.
- Top with dressing, herbs, and serve with kale and chickpeas.

Nutrition Per Serving: 247 calories| total fat 13.2 g | carbohydrates 14.2 g| protein 24 g | Cholesterol 5.3 mg| Sodium 123 mg| potassium 133 mg| Phosphorus 109 mg |Calcium 56 mg| Fiber 3.1 g

6.17 Smoked Salmon Salad with Green Dressing

Ingredients

- Smoked salmon: 180g
- Green lentils: 1/2 cup washed
- Half a cup of yogurt
- Parsley: 2 tablespoons
- Salted baby capers: 1 tablespoon
- Chives: 2 tablespoons
- Two small fennel bulbs, sliced
- Tarragon: 1 tablespoon

- Grated lemon rind: 1 teaspoon
- Half of onion, sliced
- Fresh lemon juice: 1 tablespoon
- Pinch of sugar

Instructions

- Let the lentils cook for twenty minutes or until soft, in a wide saucepan of boiling water. then drain
- In the meantime, heat a pan on high flame. Spray oil on slices of fennel. Cook per side for two minutes, or until soft.
- In a food processor, pulse the parsley, yogurt, chives, capers, tarragon, and lemon rind until creamy. season with black pepper
- In a bowl, place the sugar, onion, juice, a pinch of salt. Drain after five minutes.
- In a wide bowl, add the lentils, onion, fennel. Divide into plates. Put salmon on top. Drizzle with green dressing and fennels

Nutrition Per Serving: 310 calories| total fat 17 g | carbohydrates 12.2 g| protein 17 g | Cholesterol 5.6 mg| Sodium 141 mg| potassium 124 mg| Phosphorus 127 mg |Calcium 43 mg| Fiber 2.5 g

6.18 Greek Roasted Fish with Vegetables

Ingredients

- Four skinless salmon fillets: 5-6 ounces
- Two red, yellow, orange sweet peppers, cut into rings
- Five cloves of garlic chopped
- Sea salt: half tsp.
- Olive oil: 2 tbsp.
- Black pepper: half tsp
- Pitted halved olives: ¼ cup
- One lemon
- Parsley: 1 and ½ cups
- Finely snipped fresh oregano:1/4 cup

Instructions

- Let the oven preheat to 425 F
- Put the potatoes in a bowl. Drizzle 1 spoon of oil, sprinkle with salt (1/8 tsp.), and garlic. Mix well, shift to the baking pan, cover with foil. Roast them for half an hour
- In the meantime, thaw the salmon. Combine the sweet peppers, parsley, oregano, olives, and salt (1/8 tsp) and pepper in the same bowl. Add one tablespoon of oil, mix well.
- Wash salmon and dry it with paper towels. Sprinkle with salt (1/4 Tsp), Black pepper, and top of it, salmon. Uncover it and roast for ten minutes or till salmon starts to flake.

- Add lemon zest and lemon juice over salmon and vegetables. Serve hot

Nutrition Per Serving: 278 calories| total fat 12 g | carbohydrates 9.2 g| protein 15.4 g | Cholesterol 7.1 mg| Sodium 131 mg| potassium 141 mg| Phosphorus 121 mg |Calcium 56 mg| Fiber 3.4 g

6.19 Garlic Roasted Salmon & Brussels Sprouts

Ingredients

- Wild salmon fillet (6 portions): 2 pounds
- Olive oil: ¼ of cup
- White wine: ¾ cup
- Oregano: 2 tbsp.
- Cloves of garlic: 14
- Salt: 1 tsp.
- Lemon
- Black pepper: ¾ tsp.

Instructions:

- Let the oven pre-heat to 450 F
- take two cloves of garlic and mink them, put them in a bowl one tbsp. Of oregano, oil, half tsp. of salt and pepper (1/4 tsp.)
- In a roasting pan, halve the remaining garlic and add with Brussels sprouts and three tbsp. Of seasoned oil.
- Roast for fifteen minutes, stirring only once

- Add the wine to the remaining oil blend.
- Take out from the oven, mix vegetables, and put salmon on top.
- Sprinkle the wine oil, and salt, pepper, and oregano. Bake for ten minutes more or till fish is cooked completely. Serve with lemon.

Nutrition Per Serving: 334 calories| total fat 15.4 g | carbohydrates 10.3 g| protein 23 g | Cholesterol 6.6 mg| Sodium 134 mg| potassium 121 mg| Phosphorus 103 mg |Calcium 45 mg| Fiber 3 g

6.20 Ginger-Tahini Oven-Baked Salmon & Vegetables

Ingredients

- Salmon: 1 and ¼ pound cut into four portions
- Olive oil: two tbsp.
- Salt: half tsp.
- Light soy sauce: 2 tbsp.
- Tahini: 3 tbsp.
- Honey
- Green beans: 1 pound
- Ginger: 1 and ½ tsp.(grated)
- Chives: 2 tbsp.
- White button mushrooms: one-pound

Instructions

- Let the oven pre-heat till 425 F.

- Add a baking sheet in the range, in the upper rack, and one six inches from the broiler

- Put a broad baking sheet rimmed into the oven, place one rack in the oven center, and another about 6 inches from the broiler.

- Combine one tablespoon of oil, and mushrooms, with salt (1/4 tsp.) in a big bowl.

- Take the baking sheet out of the oven.

- Place the mixture of vegetables in one layer on the pan; start roasting it, often stirring, around 20 minutes.

- Meanwhile, mix the remaining 1 Tbsp. of oil with green beans and salt (1/4 tsp).

- In a tiny cup, mix soya sauce, ginger, tahini, and honey.

- Take out the pan from the oven. Add mushroom and sweet potatoes on one side, and on the other side place green beans.

- Place the salmon in the center. Distribute half of the tahini sauce over the salmon. Roast, for 8 to 10 minutes more, before the salmon falls.

- Switch broiler to high, transfer the pan to the top rack, and broil for around 3 minutes until the salmon is glazed.

- In the remaining tahini oil, add vinegar and drizzle over the salmon and vegetables. If needed, garnish with the chives and eat.

Nutrition Per Serving: 334 calories| total fat 13.4 g | carbohydrates 14.5 g| protein 17 g | Cholesterol 5.6 mg| Sodium 141 mg| potassium 134 mg| Phosphorus 111 mg |Calcium 56 mg| Fiber 2.7 g

6.21 Charred Shrimp & Pesto Buddha Bowls

Ingredients

- Pesto: 1/3 cup

- Vinegar: 2 tbsp.

- Olive oil: 1 tbsp.

- Salt: half tsp.

- Ground pepper: ¼ tsp.

- Peeled & deveined large shrimp: one pound

- Arugula: 4 cups

- Cooked quinoa: 2 cups

Instructions

- In a large bowl, mix pesto, oil, vinegar, salt, and pepper. Take out four tbsp. Of mixture in another bowl.

- Place skillet over medium flame. Add shrimp, let it cook for five minutes, stirring, until only charred a little. move to a plate

- Use the vinaigrette to mix with quinoa and arugula in a bowl. Divide the mixture of the arugula into four bowls. Cover with shrimp, Add 1 tbsp. Of the pesto mixture to each bowl. And serve.

Nutrition Per Serving: 329 calories| total fat 18 g | carbohydrates 17.2 g| protein 17 g | Cholesterol 6.7 mg| Sodium 154 mg| potassium 143 mg| Phosphorus 123 mg |Calcium 45 mg| Fiber 2.1 g

6.22 Salmon with Gingery Vegetables & Turmeric

Ingredients

- Salmon fillets with skin: 4pieces, 6-ounce

- Broccoli: cut into florets along with chopped stem: 1/2 pound

- Water: 3/4 cup

- Vegetable oil: 3 tablespoons

- Cauliflower, cut into florets: 1/2 pound

- One onion sliced

- Turmeric: 1/4 teaspoon

- Salt and pepper, to taste

- Soy milk: 1/2 cup

- Chopped lime pickle: 1 tablespoon

- Minced ginger: 1and 1/2 tbsp.

Instructions

- Boil broccoli and cauliflower in a deep pan, covered, for 3 minutes in half a cup of water; move to a bowl

- Heat the three tablespoons of oil in the pan. Stir in the ginger and

onion season with salt, pepper, and simmer over medium flame, stirring for around eight minutes until golden. Add the turmeric and mix until fragrant.

- Add soy milk, the pickle, and the remaining water and carry it to a simmer.

- Add the vegetables then sprinkle with salt, pepper. cover it and remove from flame

- Let the grill pan, preheat. Oil the salmon and season with salt, pepper.

- Grill, skin side down, over medium flame, for 4 minutes to crisp. Switch and grill for 2 minutes, until just cooked through. Serve the vegetables with salmon.

Nutrition Per Serving: 118 calories| total fat 6.7 g | carbohydrates 5.6 g| protein 16g | Cholesterol 8.1 mg| Sodium 123 mg| potassium 132 mg| Phosphorus 112 mg |Calcium 76 mg| Fiber 2.3 g

6.23 Simple Grilled Salmon & Vegetables

Ingredients

- Salmon fillet, cut into four portions: 1 and ¼ pounds.

- Zucchini halved lengthwise: one-piece

- Two red, orange, or yellow bell peppers: de-seeded, and halved

- One onion: cut into one wedge

- Olive oil: one tbsp.
- Salt: half tsp.
- Basil: ¼ cup
- Ground pepper: half tsp.
- Lemon into wedges

Instructions

- Let the grill pre-heat to medium-high
- Rub the onion, zucchini, and peppers with oil and salt (1/4 teaspoon).
- Sprinkle the salmon with the pepper and salt (1/4 teaspoon)
- Place the vegetables and salmon (skin side down) on the barbecue.
- Cook the vegetables, rotating once or twice, for almost five minutes per side until only soft and grill marks happen.
- Cook the salmon, without turning, for ten minutes, till it flakes.
- Cool the vegetables and Chop roughly, then put together in a dish.
- If you do not like the skin, remove it from the salmon fillets, and serve alongside the vegetables. Garnish with one tbsp. Of basil on each serving, then serve with lemon.

Nutrition Per Serving: 281 calories| total fat 12.7g | carbohydrates 10.6g|protein 20.2g | Cholesterol 7.9

mg| Sodium 154 mg| potassium 162 mg| Phosphorus 123 mg |Calcium 61 mg| Fiber 3.1 g

6.24 Broiled Salmon with Brussel sprout

Ingredients

- Steamed Brussels: 1 cup
- Fresh salmon: 4 ounces
- Light soy sauce: 2 tablespoons
- Dijon mustard: 1 and 1/2 tablespoons
- Salt & pepper, to taste

Instructions

- Let the broiler pre-heat. Cover the salmon surface with mustard and soy sauce.
- Spray the baking sheet with oil and put salmon in the baking pan, and broil for ten minutes, or until salmon completely cooked through.
- Meanwhile, steam the Brussel sprout, if not already steamed
- Serve salmon and sprinkle salt & pepper to taste.

Nutrients per serving: Calories 236|Protein 15.3 g |Carbohydrates 7.2 g| Fat 16.4 g| Cholesterol 8.9 mg| Sodium 143 mg| potassium 176 mg| Phosphorus 132 mg |Calcium 71 mg| Fiber 3 g

6.25 Zucchini Noodles with Roasted Salmon

Ingredients

- Wild Salmon: 6 ounces
- Curry paste: 1 tablespoon
- One package zucchini noodles
- Salt, pepper to taste
- Two minced cloves of garlic
- Four sliced scallions, sliced
- Half of cup of cilantro
- Two inches of ginger root(grated)
- Red pepper flakes: 1/4 teaspoon

Instructions

- Put a skillet over medium flame, and heat the coconut oil.
- Add the zoodles, curry paste, ginger and, garlic. Cook for about four minutes until the noodles are tender, keep stirring — season with Amino to taste.
- Put another skillet over medium flame and heat the coconut oil. Place skin-side down the fish. Season with red pepper flakes and salt.
- Turn on the broiler.
- Cook for seven minutes, then move to the broiler. Broil for five minutes or until the fish is completely cooked
- Add the noodles with scallions and cilantro, and stir to combine.
- Place on a plate, top with fish and serve.

Nutrients per serving: Calories 213|Protein 23.5 g |Carbohydrates 9.2 g| Fat 5.6 g| Cholesterol 13 mg| Sodium 132 mg| potassium 127 mg| Phosphorus 135 mg |Calcium 65 mg| Fiber 2.1 g

6.26 One-Sheet Roasted Garlic Salmon & Broccoli

Ingredients

- One head of broccoli cut into florets:3-4 cups
- Olive oil: 2 and 1/2 tbsp.
- Salmon fillets (4 portions): 1 1/2 pounds
- Two cloves of minced garlic
- Black pepper to taste
- Lemon slices
- Sea salt: 3/4 tsp

Instructions

- Let the oven pre-heat to 450 F and line parchment paper on baking sheet
- Put the pieces of salmon on the baking sheet, with spaces in between
- Three spray one tablespoon of oil over the fish Place the minced cloves of garlic thinly over the salmon.
- Add 1/4 teaspoon salt (or to taste) and ground black pepper to sprinkle over salmon. Finally, place the cut lemon on top of the salmon. set aside

- Then, mix 1and 1/2 tablespoons of oil, half a teaspoon of salt, and ground black pepper in a medium bowl with the broccoli florets.

- Toss the florets. Arrange the broccoli around the salmon bits into the baking dish.

- Bake in the oven for almost fifteen minutes or until fish is cooked through and the broccoli florets at the ends are slightly brown.

- Sprinkle with parsley for a garnish and, if needed, layer lemon slices around. Enjoy warm.

Nutrients per serving: Calories 256|Protein 12.3 g |Carbohydrates 9.2 g| Fat 11 g| Cholesterol 12 mg| Sodium 154 mg| potassium 187 mg| Phosphorus 145 mg |Calcium 75 mg| Fiber 2.5 g

6.27 Baked Salmon & Flaxseed Crumbs(Almonds)

Ingredients

- Salmon fillet: 1 and 1/2 pounds
- Almonds: 1/4 cup
- Bread crumbs: 1/4 cup
- Scallions, green: 1/4 cup
- Salt: 1/8 teaspoon
- Flaxseeds: 2 tablespoons
- Infused with garlic, olive oil: 1 teaspoon
- Thyme leaves: 1/4 teaspoon

- Black pepper: 1/8 teaspoon
- Lemon zest

Instructions

- Let the oven pre-heat to 450 F and line foil paper on baking sheet

- Process the flaxseeds and almonds in a mixer until a consistent, sand-like texture is obtained. take out in a bowl and add the salt, bread crumbs, pepper, scallions, thyme, lemon zest

- Put the skin-side down fish onto the baking plate. Brush the fish with oil infused with garlic, sprinkle lightly with pepper, salt. Put the crumbs on the fish evenly, and press to adhere.

- Bake fish and crumbs will turn golden brown for almost 25 minutes until it flakes easily.

Nutrients per serving: Calories 293|Protein 12 g |Carbohydrates 8.8 g| Fat 10 g| Cholesterol 9.2 mg| Sodium 123 mg| potassium 222 mg| Phosphorus 132 mg |Calcium 82.3 mg| Fiber 3.3 g

6.28 Grilled Salmon with Tartar Sauce

Ingredients

- Salmon fillets: 4 pieces
- Basil: 1/4 cup
- Garlic: Four minced
- Lemon juice: 1 cup

- Curry powder: 2 teaspoons
- Thyme: 2 teaspoons
- Butter or ghee (melted ½ cup)
- Sea salt and black pepper

Ingredients (Tartar Sauce)

- Low fat Mayonnaise: 1/2 cup
- Green onion: 1 tablespoon (chopped)
- Lemon juice: 1 tablespoon.
- Fresh dill: 1/2 teaspoon
- Mustard: 1/2 teaspoon (powder)
- Paprika: 1/4 teaspoon.
- Black pepper: 1/4 teaspoon

Instructions

- Mix the marinade ingredients in a large bowl: lemon juice, basil, garlic, curry powder, ghee, basil, thyme, sea salt, and black pepper.

- Put salmon in a see-through dish, put all the marinade on the fish and cover it. Put in the refrigerator for about 28 minutes.

- In the meantime, combine all the ingredients of the tartar sauce in a small bowl: onion, mayonnaise, lemon juice, paprika, dill, ground mustard, and black pepper. You should taste it and add any more ingredients if you desire. Please keep it in the fridge until it's time to serve.

- Now the salmon has marinated, put it on the grilling pan, and cook over medium flame and Cook for about 13 minutes.

- Pour blended sauce of tartar and enjoy.

Nutrients per serving: Calories 243|Protein 11 g |Carbohydrates 11.0 g| Fat 9 g| Cholesterol 11 mg| Sodium 132 mg| potassium 213 mg| Phosphorus 127 mg |Calcium 89.2 mg| Fiber 3 g

6.29 Oven-Fried Fish

Ingredients

- One small potato: chopped, and leahced
- Salmon filets: 4 6-ounce
- (Powder) cornmeal: ¼ cup
- Half cup minced red onion
- Lime juice: 2 tablespoons
- Salt and black pepper: ¼ teaspoon each

Instructions

- let the oven pre-heat to 400 F and spray with oil generously 2. Blend salt and pepper with cornmeal.

- Dip the fish into the cornmeal blend gently. Put on the baking sheet. Put drops of olive oil at the top of the tuna, then put it in the oven.

- Bake for 20 minutes till it is cooked.

- Mix the mashed potato with the salt, red onion, and lime juice,

- Serve the fish.

Nutrients per serving: Calories 232|Protein 11 g |Carbohydrates 12 g|

Fat 6 g| Cholesterol 22 mg| Sodium 132 mg| potassium 213 mg| Phosphorus 132 mg |Calcium 78 mg| Fiber 2.3 g

6.30 Fish Tacos

Ingredients

- Cabbage: 1-1/2 cups
- Half cup red onion
- Half bunch of cilantro
- 1 garlic clove
- Two limes
- Tuna fillets: 4 cups
- Sour cream: 1/4 cup
- Half tsp. Of ground cumin
- Half tsp. Of chili powder
- Soy milk: 2 tablespoons
- Black pepper: 1/4 teaspoon
- Olive oil: 1 tablespoon
- 1/2 cup mayonnaise (low fat)-optional
- 12 flour tortillas

Instructions

- Chop up the cilantro and onion, and Shred the cabbage
- Marinate the fish in lime juice, minced garlic, black pepper, olive oil, chili powder, cumin. Mix well and chill in the fridge for half an hour.
- Make the salsa by mixing sour cream, milk, lime juice, and mayonnaise. Mix well and set it aside in the refrigerator
- Let the oven on to broil, lay the foil on the broiler pan.
- Broil the marinated fish until it turns white and flakes easily, for ten minutes.
- Take out from oven, flake fish into pieces.
- Warm up the tortillas.
- Top tortilla with fish flakes, salsa, red onion, cabbage.
- Serve right away and enjoy

Nutrients per serving: Calories 363|Protein 18 g |Carbohydrates 30 g|

Fat 19 g|Cholesterol 40 mg|Sodium 194 mg|potassium 507 mg|Phosphorus 327 mg |Calcium 138 mg|Fiber 4.3 g

6.31 Creamy fish and Broccoli Fettuccine

Ingredients

- Ground peppercorns: 3/4 teaspoon
- Half cup of fettuccine, uncooked
- One cup fresh fish
- Nondairy creamer: 1/4 cup
- Two cloves of garlic
- Broccoli florets: 1-3 cup
- Lemon juice: 1/4 cup
- Red bell pepper: 1/4 cup

- One cup of cream cheese (low fat)

Instructions

- Cook pasta to your liking without salt.

- Add the floret of broccoli in the last three minutes of pasta cooking.

- Over medium flame, in a pan, stir garlic and fish for 2 to 3 minutes. Add lemon juice, cream cheese, creamer and, ground peppercorns—Cook for two more minutes.

- Add pasta and mix with the fish mix. Add in the bell pepper.

Nutrients per serving: calories 448 |Protein 27 g| Carbohydrates 28 g| Fat 28 g| Cholesterol 203 mg| Sodium 364 mg| Potassium 369 mg| Phosphorus 315 mg| Calcium 157 mg| Fiber 2.6 g

6.32 Creamy Baked Fish

Ingredients

- All-purpose white flour: half cup

- One pound of fish (your choice)

- Salt: 1/4 teaspoon

- Pepper: 1/4 teaspoon

- Non-dairy creamer(fat-free): one cup

- Unsalted butter: 2 tablespoons

- Water: 1/4 cup

- Non-dairy creamer(regular): 1 cup

Instructions

- Let the oven preheat to 350 F

- Take an 8 by 8 baking glass dish, spray with cooking oil. Coat the dish lightly with flour.

- Place fish fillets in the dish and add pepper, salt, and flour on top.

- Pour non-dairy creamers and water on fish

- Add butter pieces on top.

- Bake for half an hour to 45 minutes or until golden brown.

- Serve with creamy sauce.

Nutrients per serving: Calories 380|Protein 23 g| Carbohydrates 46 g| Fat 11 g| Cholesterol 79 mg| Sodium 253 mg| Potassium 400 mg| Phosphorus 266 mg| Calcium 46 mg| Fiber 0.4 g

6.33 Tasty Baked Fish

Ingredients

- Olive oil: 2 tablespoons

- Half tsp. Of ground cumin

- Half tsp. Of black pepper

- One pound of any fish fillets

- Half tsp. of ground rosemary

Instructions

- Let the oven preheat to 350 F.

- Pour olive oil on fish and coat well

- Add spices over fish.

- Put in a baking dish.
- Bake for 20-25 minutes or until completely cooked through
- Serve hot

Nutrients per serving: Calories 171| Protein 20 g| Carbohydrates 0 g| Fat 10 g| Cholesterol 68 mg| Sodium 69 mg| Potassium 338 mg| Phosphorus 204 mg| Calcium 39 mg|Fiber 0.2 g

6.34 Crunchy Oven-Fried Catfish

Ingredients

- Catfish fillets: 1 pound
- One egg white
- Cornmeal: 1/4 cup
- Panko bread crumbs: 1/4 cup
- Half cup all-purpose flour
- Cajun seasoning(salt-free): 1 teaspoon

Instructions

- Let the oven preheat to 450 F.
- Spray oil on a baking tray.
- In a mixer, whisk the egg until soft peak forms.
- Add flour on a parchment paper. On another sheet of parchment, mix the Cajun seasoning, cornmeal, and panko.
- Slice the fish into four fillets.
- Coat the fillet in flour, then in egg white, then in cornmeal mix.

- Dip the fish in the flour and shake off excess.
- Place the coated fish on a baking pan.
- Spray the fish fillets with cooking spray.
- Bake for 10 to 12 minutes, turn the fish over, and bake for another five minutes.
- Serve hot

Nutrients per serving: Calories 250| Protein 22 g| Carbohydrates 19 g| Fat 10 g| Cholesterol 53 mg| Sodium 124 mg| Potassium 401 mg| Phosphorus 262 mg| Calcium 26 mg| Fiber 1.2 g

6.35 Salmon with Lemon Caper Sauce

Ingredients

- Cooked white rice: 4-1/2 cups
- Raw tuna steaks: 20 ounces
- Lemon juice: 4 tablespoons
- White wine: 1/4 cup
- Olive oil: 1 tablespoon
- All-purpose white flour: 2 teaspoons
- White pepper: 1/4 teaspoon
- Half cup of chicken broth reduced-sodium
- Unsalted butter: 2 tablespoons
- Capers: 1 teaspoon

Instructions

- In a zip lock bag, add olive oil, two tablespoons of lemon juice. Add fish in zip lock bag marinate for five minutes.

- Spray oil on a skillet over medium flame, cook the fish for three minutes.

- Flip the fish and cook for two minutes more.

- In a skillet, melt butter, add flour, and mix. Add broth cook for one minute.

- Add remaining lemon juice, pepper, wine, and capers. Continue to mix and cook for five minutes or until sauce thickens.

- Serve fish with rice and caper sauce.

Nutrients per serving: Calories 340| Protein 26 g| Carbohydrates 34 g| Fat 9 g| Cholesterol 46 mg| Sodium 118 mg| Potassium 573 mg| Phosphorus 306 mg| Calcium 79 mg| Fiber 0.6 g

6.36 Mango Ginger Mahi Mahi

Ingredients

- Mahi-mahi fillets: 1-1/2 pounds

- Sweet mango chutney: 1/2 cup

- 2 tbsp. Of vinegar

- Gingerroot: 1 tablespoon minced

- Soy sauce(reduced-sodium): 2 tablespoons

- One clove of minced garlic

- Olive oil: 2 tablespoons

- White pepper: 1 teaspoon

Instructions

- Mix all ingredients, and pour over fish.

- Chill in the fridge for 20 minutes at least

- In a pan, spray oil, and cook fish skin side down

- Cook for 4-6 minutes over medium-low heat, on each side, turn only once.

- In a pan, reduce the leftover marinade and pour over fish and Serve hot

Nutrients per serving: Calories 221 | Protein 21 g |Carbohydrates 9 g| Fat 10 g| Cholesterol 80 mg| Sodium 298 mg| Potassium 547 mg| Phosphorus 175 mg| Calcium 27 mg| Fiber 0.6 g

6.37 Grilled Salmon

Ingredients

- Salmon fillets: 1 pound

- Lemon juice: 1/4 cup

- Lemon pepper salt-free seasoning: 1 teaspoon

Instructions

- Sprinkle the salmon with seasoning. Pour lemon juice over the top. Spray with oil.

- Put on pre heated grill

- cook for 15 to 20 minutes or until cooked through.

- Serve hot.

Nutrients per serving: Calories 161| Protein 23 g| Carbohydrates 0 g| Fat 8 g| Cholesterol 63 mg| Sodium 49 mg| Potassium 556 mg| phosphorus 227 mg| Calcium 15 mg|Fiber 0 g

6.38 Grilled Blackened Tilapia

Ingredients

- Olive oil: 2 tablespoons
- Four tilapia filets
- Dried oregano: 1 teaspoon
- Half teaspoon. Of cayenne pepper
- 2 cloves of minced garlic
- Smoked paprika: 2 teaspoons
- Cumin: 3/4 teaspoon.

Instructions

- Preheat the grill on medium heat spray oil on the grill.
- Mix all the seasoning and coat the fish.
- Grill for almost three minutes on each side, or until cooked through
- Top with cilantro and serve

Nutrition per serving: Total Fat 9.3g| Cholesterol 58mg| Sodium 62.4mg| Total Carbohydrate 1.8g| Dietary Fiber 0.8g| Protein 23.7g| Iron 1.4mg| Potassium 403mg| Phosphorus 207.3mg|

6.39 Zesty Orange Tilapia

Ingredients

- Zest orange peel: 2 teaspoons

- Tilapia: 16 ounces
- Celery: ¾ cup, julien cut
- Ground black pepper: 1 teaspoon
- Half cup of sliced green onions
- Orange juice: 4 teaspoons
- Carrots: 1 cup, Julien cut

Instructions

- Let the oven preheat to 450° F.
- In a bowl, mix green onions, orange zest, carrots, celery.
- Slice the fish into four equal parts. Spray oil on four large squares of foil.
- Add ¼ of vegetables in each foil square, then add fish on top.
- Add black pepper and one tsp. of orange juice on top.
- Cover with foil and fold edges make a pouch.
- Bake for about 12 minutes or more if required.
- Serve in foil.

Nutrition Per Serving: calories 133 | Total Fat 2 g| Saturated Fat 1 g| Trans Fat 0 g| Cholesterol 57 mg| Sodium 97 mg| Carbohydrates 6 g| Protein 24 g| Phosphorus 214 mg| Potassium 543 mg| Dietary Fiber 1.7 g

Calcium 42 mg

6.40 Pesto-Crusted Catfish

Ingredients

- Pesto: 4 teaspoons

- Catfish: 2 pounds (no bones)
- Panko bread crumbs: ¾ cup
- Olive oil: 2 tablespoons
- Half cup of vegan cheese
- Seasoning Blend: (No salt added spices)
- Red pepper flakes: half teaspoon
- Garlic powder: 1 teaspoon
- Dried oregano: half teaspoon
- Black pepper: half teaspoon
- Onion powder: 1 teaspoon

Instructions

- Let the oven preheat to 400 F
- In a bowl, add all the seasoning, sprinkle over fish, both sides.
- Then spread pesto on each side of fish
- In a bowl, mix bread crumbs, cheese, oil. Coat pesto fish in crumbs mix.
- Spray oil on the baking tray. Add fish on a baking tray.
- Bake at 400° F for 20 minutes or until you want.
- Let it rest for ten minutes. Then serve

Nutrition Per Serving: Calories 312 | total Fat 16 g |Saturated Fat 3 g| Trans Fat 0 mg| Cholesterol 83 mg| Sodium 272 mg| Carbohydrates 15 g| Protein 26 g| Phosphorus 417 mg| Potassium 576 mg| Dietary Fiber 0.8 g| Calcium 80 mg

6.41 Citrus Salmon

Ingredients

- Salmon filet: 24 ounces
- Olive oil: 2 tablespoons
- Dijon mustard: 1 tablespoon
- Two garlic cloves, minced
- Dried basil leaves: 1 teaspoon
- Lemon juice: 1-1/2 tbsp.
- Unsalted butter: 1 tablespoon
- Cayenne pepper: 2 pinches
- Capers: 1 tablespoon
- Dried dill: 1 teaspoon

Instructions

- In a pan, add all the ingredients but do not add salmon. Let it boil, then lower the flame and cook for five minutes.
- Preheat the grill. Put the fish on a large piece of foil, skin side down.
- Fold the edges. Put the fish in foil on the grill. Add sauce over the salmon
- Cover the grill, let it cook for 12 minutes, do not flip the fish.
- Serve hot

Nutrients per serving: Calories 294| Protein 23 g| Carbohydrates 1 g| Fat 22 g| Cholesterol 68 mg| Sodium 190 mg| Potassium 439 mg| Phosphorus 280 mg | Calcium 21 mg| Fiber 0.2 g

6.42 Adobo-Marinated Tilapia Tapas

Ingredients

- Six pieces of tilapia filets
- Small wonton: 48 wrappers

Slaw Mix

- Green scallions: ¼ cup, thinly sliced
- Half cup of low-fat mayonnaise
- Fresh cabbage: 4 cups
- Lemon juice: ¼ cup
- Fresh garlic: 1 tablespoon, chopped
- Cilantro leaves: ¼ cup, roughly chopped

Adobo Sauce

- Oregano: 1 tablespoon
- Spanish paprika: 3 tablespoons
- Extra-virgin olive oil: ¼ cup
- Fresh cilantro: 3 tablespoons chopped
- Red pepper flakes: 1 teaspoon
- Half cup of red wine vinegar
- Black pepper: 1 teaspoon

Instructions

- Let the oven preheat to 400° F.
- In a bowl, mix adobo ingredients and set it aside
- Marinate the fish filets in half a cup of adobe sauce for half an hour.
- Spray oil on a baking tray and bake the fish for 15 minutes. Halfway through, flip the fish. Take out from the oven and set it aside.
- In a bowl, add claw slaw ingredients and mix well.
- Spray the oil over the muffin pan. Add one wonton wrapper in muffin cups.
- Bake for five minutes at 350 F, and then cool the crispy wontons
- Add fish in crispy wonton top with slaw mix. Top with cilantro leaves.

Nutrition Per Serving: Calories 254| Total Fat 13 g| saturated Fat 2 g| Trans Fat 0 g| Cholesterol 28 mg| Sodium 272 mg| Carbohydrates 22 g| protein 13 g | phosphorus 116 mg| Potassium 268 mg|dietary Fiber 2 g| Calcium 46 mg

6.43 Fiesta Tilapia Ceviche

Ingredients

- Chopped half cup of red bell pepper
- Fresh tilapia fillets: 1 and 1/2 pounds, cut into cubes
- Chopped red onion: 1 cup
- Chopped cilantro: 1/4 cup
- Olive oil: 2 tablespoons
- Fresh lime juice: 1-1/4 cups
- Pineapple: 1 cup
- Unsalted crackers
- Black pepper: 1/4 teaspoon

Instructions

- For three minutes, broil the fish cubes on each side

- Pour lime juice over broiled fish (cool it first for five minutes). Mix well

- Mix the oil, onion, pineapple, bell pepper, black pepper, cilantro. And pour overcooked fish.

- Let it marinate for two hours or more in the fridge

- Serve fish with unsalted crackers.

Nutrients per serving: Calories 220| Protein 19 g| Carbohydrates 20 g| Fat 7 g| Cholesterol 36 mg| sodium 168 mg| Potassium 374 mg| Phosphorus 162 mg| Calcium 43 mg| Fiber 1.3 g

6.44 Korean-Style Fried White Fish

Ingredients

- All-purpose white flour: 3 tablespoons

- Unseasoned rice vinegar: 1 tablespoon

- White fish fillets: 1 pound

- Reduced-sodium soy sauce: 1 teaspoon

- Two large egg whites whisked

- Sesame oil: 3 tablespoons

- Half tsp. of black pepper

Instructions

- In a bowl, mix soy sauce with vinegar.

- Cut the fish into one and a half-inch pieces.

- In a zip lock bag, add pepper and flour, add the fish in bag and coat well

- in a skillet heat the sesame oil, coat the flour-coated fish into eggs. Fry in hot oil until golden brown.

- Serve hot.

Nutrients per serving: Calories 273 | Protein 26 g| Carbohydrates 4 g| Fat 17 g| Cholesterol 151 mg| Sodium 134 mg| Potassium 400 mg| Phosphorus 359 mg| Calcium 42 mg| Fiber 0.1 g

6.45 Sole with Tarragon Cream Sauce

Ingredients

- Sole fillets: 1 pound

- Sliced green onions: 1/4 cup

- One clove of minced garlic

- Sliced green olives: 2 tablespoons

- Dried tarragon: 1 teaspoon

- Olive oil: 2 tablespoons

- Fresh lemon juice: 1/4 cup

- Sour cream: 1/3 cup

- Dried basil: 1/2 teaspoon

Instructions

- Sauté garlic and onion in olive oil till tender

- Add in the lemon juice, herbs, sour cream, olives.

- Mix well and heat for one minute. Turn off the heat and set it aside.

- In a microwave-proof dish, add the roll up the fish fillet, with a toothpick secure it.

- Add sauce to the fish, microwave for four minutes.

- Take out the toothpicks, serve with sauce.

Nutrients per serving: calories 216| Protein 22 g| Carbohydrates 3 g|Fat 12 g| Cholesterol 65 mg| Sodium 188 mg| Potassium 388 mg| Phosphorus 269 mg| Calcium 52 mg|Fiber 0.3 g

6.46 Eggplant Seafood Casserole

- Ingredients
- 3 eggs' white
- Eggplants: 2 medium
- One onion
- Half cup of celery
- Two garlic cloves
- Worcestershire: 1 tablespoon
- Olive oil: 1/4 cup
- One bell pepper
- Lemon juice: 1/4 cup
- Creole seasoning: 1/4 teaspoon
- Half tsp. Of tabasco
- Rice: 1/3 cup, uncooked

- Lump crab meat: 1 pound
- Unsalted butter: 2 tablespoons, melted
- Half pound boiled fish
- Half cup bread crumbs
- vegan cheese: 1/4 cup

Instructions

- Let the oven preheat to 350 F
- Chop up the celery, onion, and bell pepper.
- Dice and peel the eggplant into one-inch cubes.
- Boil eggplant for five minutes until tender, drain the water, and set it aside
- In olive oil, sauté celery, garlic, bell pepper, and onion, do not let them brown
- In a bowl, add eggplant, sautéed vegetables, Creole seasonings, lemon juice, Tabasco sauce, Worcestershire sauce, eggs, cayenne, rice, and cheese. Mix well
- Add seafood to the vegetable mix. Put in a casserole dish, oil the dish well before.
- Mix melted butter with bread crumbs and add on top of casserole.
- Bake for half an hour or until topping begins to brown.

Nutrients per serving: Calories 216 | Protein 13 g| Carbohydrates 14 g| Fat 12 g |Cholesterol 138 mg| Sodium 229 mg| Potassium 359 mg| Phosphorus 148 mg |Calcium 79 mg| Fiber 2.3 g

6.47 Honey Spice-Rubbed Salmon

Ingredients

- 16 ounces of salmon fillets
- Honey: 3 tablespoons
- Half tsp. Of black pepper
- 2 pressed cloves of garlic
- Lemon peel: 3/4 teaspoon
- Hot water: 1 teaspoon
- Arugula: 3 cups
- Olive oil: 2 tablespoons

Instructions

- In a bowl, add grated lemon peel, honey, hot water, ground pepper, garlic, and whisk well.
- With clean hands, rub the mixture over fish fillets.
- Over medium flame, heat the olive oil in a pan. Add marinated fish fillets and cook for four minutes. Turn once.
- Turn the heat to low and cook for 4-6 minutes or until fish is cooked through.
- Add half a cup of arugula to the plate. Put salmon fillet on arugula.
- Sprinkle with fresh herbs and serve.

Nutrients per serving: Calories 323 | Protein 23 g |Carbohydrates 15 g| Fat

19 g| Cholesterol 62 mg| Sodium 66 mg| Potassium 454 mg| Phosphorus 261 mg| Calcium 42 mg|Fiber 0.4 g

6.48 Cilantro-Lime swordfish

Ingredients

- Swordfish: 1 pound
- Half cup of low-fat mayonnaise
- Lime juice: 2 tablespoon
- Half cup of fresh cilantro

Instructions

- In a bowl, mix chopped cilantro, lime juice, low-fat mayonnaise, mix well.
- Take ¼ cup from the mix and leave the rest aside
- Apply the rest of the mayo mix to the fish with a brush
- In a skillet, over medium heat, spray oil
- Add fish fillets, cook for 8 minutes, turning once, or until fish is cooked to your liking.
- Serve with sauce.

Nutrients per serving: Calories 292 | Protein 20 g |Carbohydrates 1 g| Fat 23 g| Cholesterol 57 mg| Sodium 228 mg| Potassium 237 mg| Phosphorus 128 mg| Calcium 14 mg| Fiber 0 g

6.49 Grilled Mexican Swordfish Fillets

Ingredients

- Olive oil: 1 tablespoon

- Swordfish fillets: 1 and 1/2 pounds'
- Lime juice: 1/4 cup
- Fresh cilantro: 1/4 cup
- Onion: 1/4 cup
- One tablespoon honey
- Salt: 1/4 teaspoon
- One serrano chili
- One lime
- Two cloves of garlic

Instructions

- Finely dice the onion and chili (seeded).
- Place swordfish in a baking dish
- In a food blender, mix cilantro, honey, salt (1/4 tsp.), onion, garlic, oil, and lime juice. Pulse until smooth.
- Pour this mix over fish, coat the fish well, let it marinate in the fridge for half an hour.
- Let the grill preheat.
- Grill for five minutes on every side, or fish is completely cooked through.
- Serve with lime wedges and enjoy.

Nutrients per serving: Calories 198|Protein 23 g| Carbohydrates 4 g| Fat 10 g| Cholesterol 75 mg| Sodium 190 mg| Potassium 506 mg| Phosphorus 295 mg |Calcium 11 mg| Fiber 0.2 g

6.50 Lemon Pepper Salmon

- Extra virgin olive oil: 2 tablespoons
- Salmon: 2 pounds, boneless (skin on or off)
- Ten sprigs of thyme
- Chopped fresh herbs of your choice
- Kosher salt: 1 teaspoon
- Black pepper: 1/2 teaspoon
- Two medium lemons

Instructions

- Let the oven preheat to 375 F.
- Place aluminum foil over a baking tray or parchment paper
- Spray oil over the foil, place five sprigs of thyme in the middle. Add lemon slices over the thyme. Add the fish on top.
- Add zest, olive oil, salt, and pepper over fish.
- Add the remaining thyme and lemon slices and lemon juice on top of the fish.
- Pack the salmon in foil, completely closed, leave some room in the foil.
- Bake for 15-19 minutes or until salmon is cooked.
- When salmon is cooked, uncover it and let it broil for three minutes.
- Do not overcook the salmon.

- Serve with fresh lemon juice and herbs on top.

Nutrition per serving: calories 268kcal| carbohydrates: 4g|protein: 31g| fat: 14g| saturated fat: 2g| cholesterol: 83mg |potassium: 801mg| fiber: 1g|sugar: 1g| calcium: 34mg|iron: 2mg

6.51 Easy Salmon Soup

- Salmon fillet without skin: 1 lb.
- Extra virgin olive oil
- Half chopped green bell pepper
- Chicken broth(low-sodium): 5 cups
- Four cloves of minced garlic
- Four diced green onions
- 2 tbsp. Of dill chopped
- Dry oregano: 1 tsp
- One cup of potatoes(leached), thinly sliced
- One carrot cut into thinly sliced
- Ground coriander: ¾ tsp
- Salt and black pepper
- Juice and zest of one lemon
- Half tsp of ground cumin

Instructions

- In a large pot, heat two tablespoons of oil, add garlic, bell pepper, green onions, cook over medium flame. Stir often.
- Add half of the dill, and cook for 30 seconds.
- Add chicken broth, carrots, and potatoes.
- Add black pepper, spices, and salt. Let it boil, lower the heat and cook for five minutes to make sure they are tender.
- Add salt to salmon and add in the soup. Lower the heat and cook for few minutes until salmon is cooked and will flake easily.
- Add in lemon juice, zest, and dill.
- Serve hot.

Nutrients per serving: Calories 218|Protein 24 g| Carbohydrates 3.3 g| Fat 8.9 g| Cholesterol 68 mg| Sodium 181 mg| Potassium 232 mg| Phosphorus 213 mg |Calcium 9.9 mg| Fiber 8 g

Chapter 7: Kidney-Friendly Vegetables Recipes

7.1 Vegan Lettuce Wrap Recipe

Ingredients

- 2 cups of extra firm tofu
- ¼ cup of dry white rice
- Butter lettuce: 4 medium leaves
- One clove of pressed garlic
- Honey: 2 teaspoons
- 1 teaspoon of freshly grated ginger
- Cauliflower: 1 cup
- Low sodium soy sauce: 1 tablespoon
- Rice vinegar: 2 tablespoons
- Olive oil: 1 tablespoon
- Sesame oil: 1 tablespoon
- Half cup of shredded carrots

Instructions

- Let the oven Pre-heat to 400F.
- Cook the rice as you want, but do not add butter or salt.
- Cut the cauliflower in very small pieces like rice grain size.
- A small food processor mix ginger, garlic, honey, rice vinegar, soy sauce, sesame oil.
- Cut the tofu into bite-size. Spray olive oil on tofu and bake at 400F for 20 minutes' flip halfway through.
- Mix the chopped up cauliflower with freshly cooked rice.
- Toss the tofu with a sauce prepared earlier.
- Lay lettuce leaves on a flat surface, top with cauliflower/rice mix and the sauce, then tofu.

Nutrition per serving: Calories 410| Total Fat 26g| Saturated Fat 4g| Cholesterol 0mg| Sodium 187mg|Total Carbohydrate 34g| Dietary Fiber 4g| Total Sugars 9g|Protein 14g, Calcium 148mg| Iron 3mg| Potassium 441mg

7.2 Vegan Bell Pepper, Kidney Bean, & Cilantro Salad

Ingredients

- 1 tablespoon of extra virgin olive oil
- Half cup diced cilantro
- 2-3 cloves of pressed garlic
- 2 cups of red bell pepper diced
- ¼ cup of chopped macadamia nuts or walnuts
- One can chickpeas or kidney beans
- Salt, pepper to taste

Instructions

- In a big bowl, add all ingredients. Mix them well.
- Season with salt and freshly ground black pepper.

- Garnish with olive oil.

Nutrition per serving: Calories 105, Fat 9g, Sodium 8 mg, Potassium 125 mg, Carbohydrates 4g, Fiber 1g, Protein 2g, Calcium 40mg, Iron 1.4mg8%

7.3 Vegetable Paella

Ingredients

- White rice: 2 cups, uncooked
- Green beans: one and a half cups
- Olive oil: 1 tablespoon
- Green bell pepper chopped: 1 cup
- broccoli florets: 3 cups
- 1 cup of diced zucchini
- Half cup of chopped onion
- Half tsp. of salt

Instructions

- Cook rice to your preference without salt and butter.
- Add broccoli and green beans in a saucepan, add water to cover them.
- Let them boil for four minutes and drain
- In a pan, heat oil over medium flame. Sauté the broccoli, zucchini, onion, beans, and bell pepper, cook for 4-5 minutes.
- Add in the remaining ingredients. Cook for five minutes, stirring frequently.

Nutrients per serving: Calories 146, Protein 5 g, Carbohydrates 26 g, Fat 2

g, Cholesterol 0 mg, Sodium 150 mg, Potassium 305 mg, Phosphorus 89 mg, Calcium 38 mg, Fiber 1.8 g

7.4 Broccoli & Mushrooms with Sweet Potatoes

Ingredients

- Four medium-sized baked sweet potatoes
- Two tablespoons of olive oil
- 2 cups of mushrooms, sliced
- 1 head of broccoli, cut into tiny florets
- 1/3 cup broth, hot, low-sodium (veggie)
- Black pepper fresh ground, to taste
- 2/3 cup basic, low-fat yogurt

Instructions

- Make sure that the potatoes are entirely dry—dust one tablespoon of olive oil with the potatoes. Wrap Every potato in aluminum foil. Put in a slow cooker, seal, and cook for 7-8 hours at the low flame or 4-5 hours at high heat until the potatoes are tender.
- On medium flame, heat the remaining tbsp. of olive oil in a large pan. Add the mushrooms & broccoli and sauté for around ten minutes till the broccoli is tender but not soft.
- Unpack the foil from each potato. Create a slice of potatoes in

the center and scrape the potato into a pan. Add broth, yogurt, and pepper. Blend to mix. Split it up back into the potato skins and stuff. Cover it with mushrooms and broccoli.

Nutrition per serving: Calories: 330, Total Fat: 7 g, Sodium: 360 mg, Total Carbs: 57 g, Dietary Fiber: 8 g, Protein: 14 g, potassium 234 mg, phosphorous 66 mg

7.5 Mediterranean Stew with Vegetables

Ingredients

- 1 sweet potato, trimmed and cut into cubes (leached)
- 1 cubed eggplant
- One big, cut into cubes zucchini
- 1 medium yellow onion, chopped
- 1 onion, sliced
- 1 carrot, finely chopped
- 2 garlic cloves, chopped up
- 1 cup of no sodium tomato sauce (homemade)
- 1/2 cup broth of vegetables, no sodium
- 1/2 teaspoon cumin ground
- 1/2 of a teaspoon of turmeric
- 1/2 teaspoon of red pepper crushed
- ¼ tsp. of the paprika

Instructions

- Add all the ingredients in a slow cooker. Mash, cover, and cook for 7-8 hours on low or 4-5 hours on high, just until the veggies are tender.
- Serve hot.

Nutrition per serving: Calories: 122| Total Fat: .5 g| Sodium: 157 mg| Total Carbs: 30 g| Dietary Fiber: 7.8 g |Protein: 3.4 g| potassium 176 mg|phosphorous 89 mg

7.6 Florentine Mushroom

Ingredients

- Half cup of whole-grain pasta
- 1/4 cup no sodium broth
- 1 cup of sliced mushrooms
- 1/4 cup of milk soybeans
- Olive oil for 1 teaspoon
- 1/2 teaspoon of Italian seasonings

Instructions

- Cook the pasta as per the direction.
- Add in the saucepan with olive oil and heat up.
- Add Italian seasonings and mushrooms. Mix well and cook for ten minutes.
- Then incorporate chicken stock and soy milk.
- Shake the combination well enough and add the cooked pasta. Cook it over low heat for 5 minutes.

Nutrition per serving: 287 calories| 12.4g protein| 20.4g carbohydrates| 4.2g fat| 9g fiber| 0mg cholesterol| potassium 123 m| phosphorus 111 mg

7.7 Bean Hummus

Ingredients

- 1 cup of soaked chickpeas
- Six Cups of Water
- 1 tbsp. of tahini paste
- Two cloves of garlic,
- Olive oil: 1/4 cup
- 1/4 Cup of Lemon Juice
- One Harissa tsp.

Instructions

- In the saucepan, add water. Add chickpeas, then close the cover.
- On the low temperature, cook the chickpeas for 40 minutes or once they're soft.
- Move the cooked chickpeas into the mixing bowl after this.
- Garnish with olive oil, lemon juice, harissa, cloves of garlic, and tahini Paste.
- Until it's smooth, mix the hummus.

Nutrition per serving: 215 calories, 7.1g protein, 21.6g carbohydrates, 12g fat, 6.1g fiber, potassium 135 mg, phosphorous 126 mg

7.8 Hassel Back Eggplant

Ingredients

- Two eggplants
- Two red peppers, sliced together
- 1 tbsp. of yogurt with low fat
- 1 tsp of powdered curry
- Olive oil for 1 teaspoon

Instructions

- Make cuts in the form of the Hassel back in the eggplants.
- Then add the curry powder on the vegetables and fill them with sliced tomatoes.
- Spray the olive oil and yogurt on the eggplants and cover them in the foil (cover each Hassel back eggplant individually).
- For 25 minutes, cook the vegetables at 375F.

Nutrition per serving: 188 calories, 7g protein, 38.1g carbohydrates, 3g fat, 21.2g fiber, Potassium 99.9 mg, phosphorous 87 mg

7.9 Roasted Cauliflower & Turmeric Curry

Ingredients

Masala

- Half cup of raw cashews
- Coriander seeds: 1 and 1/2 tablespoons
- Cardamom powder: a pinch
- Cumin seeds: 1 teaspoon
- One and 1/4-inch of cinnamon stick

- Six cloves of garlic

Curry

- Half tsp. of salt
- Turmeric powder: 1 teaspoon
- Olive oil: 2 tablespoons
- Three cloves of pressed garlic
- One cm of grated fresh ginger root
- Cauliflower florets: 2 cups
- Soy milk: 2 cups
- One chopped capsicum or bell pepper
- Red onions: 2 cups, finely chopped
- Roma tomatoes: half of a cup, finely chopped
- Half teaspoon of chili powder
- One teaspoon of Himalayan salt
- One and a 1/2 cups water
- Chopped coriander: 1 tablespoon (cilantro)
- Half teaspoon of garam masala

Instructions

Turmeric Roasted Cauliflower

- Let the oven preheat to 400 F
- In a big bowl, add the cauliflower, pinch of salt, coconut oil, and powdered turmeric, with your clean hands' mix and rub on cauliflower.

- Line a baking tray with parchment paper and pour this mixture in it and bake in the oven for half an hour. Check often to make sure cauliflower does not burn.
- Little roasted should be fine. Make sure not to overcook it.

The Curry

- In the meantime, as cauliflower is roasting.
- In a food processor bowl, add all the masala ingredients, pulse on high until completely smooth. Make sure no lumps remain.
- In a pan, over low heat, melt the coconut oil and stir in the ginger, garlic, onions and cook carefully for three minutes.
- Then add the chopped bell pepper, the tomatoes, until tomatoes are melted and falling apart.
- Add in the masala mix and stir for 2-3 minutes, do not let it burn or stick to the pan.
- When the mixture is well-combined, add in the chili powder, turmeric, and coconut milk. Add as much water as needed to get the desired consistency.
- Turn the flame down to low, let it simmer, and cook for five minutes. Adjust seasoning, and cauliflower will be ready by then, add into the pan.
- Mix well and turn off the flame. Top with cilantro and serve hot.

- It tastes well with rice or quinoa.

Nutrition per serving: Calories: 163.2, Total Fat 14.2 g, Saturated Fat 2 g, Cholesterol 0 mg, Sodium 126.7 mg, Total Carbohydrate 8.6 g, Dietary Fiber 3.5 g, Sugars 1.9 g, Protein 3 g, Potassium 187 mg, phosphorous 121 mg

7.10 One-Pot Zucchini Mushroom Pasta

Ingredients

- Two zucchinis, quartered and thinly sliced

- Grain spelt or Kamut spaghetti: 4 cups

- Two sprigs of thyme

- Walnut milk: 1/4 cup(homemade)

- Cayenne pepper and Sea salt to taste

- Cremini mushrooms: 4 cups, thinly sliced

Instructions

- In a big pot, add mushrooms, thyme, zucchini, and spaghetti with 4 and 1/2 cup of water, over medium flame. Season according to taste with cayenne pepper and sea salt.

- Let it boil, then lower the flame and let it simmer, do not cover. Let the pasta cook for ten minutes, until liquid has significantly reduced.

- Add in the milk.

- Top with cilantro and Serve hot. Enjoy.

Nutrition per serving: Calories 378.7, Total Fat 6.5g, Saturated Fat 3.4g, Trans Fat 0g, Cholesterol 17.6mg, Sodium 109.3mg, Total Carbohydrate 64.8g, Dietary Fiber 4.3g, Sugars 5.8g, Protein 15.8g, Potassium 145 mg, phosphorous 92.3 mg

7.11 Quinoa Stuffed Spaghetti Squash

Ingredients

- Two tbsp. of coconut oil

- Green peas(steamed): 1 cup

- One shallot (medium)

- One red or orange bell pepper

- Two spring of green onions, thinly sliced white part

- Cooked quinoa: 1 and 1/2 cup

- Chopped walnuts: 1/4 cup

- Two smaller or one big spaghetti squashes

- One tsp. of garlic powder

- Two tsp. of dried thyme

- Black pepper and Pink salt to taste

Instructions

- Let the oven preheat to 400 F

- Wash and pat dry the squash and half them. Take out the seeds and bake for 40 minutes. Until tender

- In a pan, add one tbsp. Of oil and add the bell pepper, shallots. Cook until tender.

- Add cooked quinoa, spices and green peas, and walnuts—season with black pepper and salt.

- Cut the squash in further half and bake for another five to 8 minutes. Take out the squash from the oven and with a fork, scratch it until resembles spaghetti.

- Serve with the vegetable mixture.

Nutrition per serving: Calories: 108kcal | Carbohydrates: 20g | Protein: 3g | Fat: 1g | Sodium: 132mg | Potassium: 251mg | Fiber: 3g | Sugar: 3g | Calcium: 29mg | Iron: 1.3mg

7.12 Kale Pesto Pasta

Ingredients

- One spiralized zucchini(zoodles)
- One bunch of kale
- Extra virgin olive oil: 1/4 cup
- Half cup of walnuts
- Fresh basil: 2 cups
- Fresh-squeezed: 2 limes
- Garnish with tomato, and beans
- Sea salt and pepper, to taste

Instructions

- Soak walnuts, overnight.
- Add all ingredients in a food blender.

- Pulse on high and smooth and creamy. Add this sauce over zucchini noodles

- Serve and enjoy.

Nutrition per serving: Calories: 108kcal | Carbohydrates: 10g | Protein: 3g | Fat: 0.8 g | Sodium: 102mg | Potassium: 131mg | Fiber: 3g | Sugar: 1.9 g | Calcium: 32 mg | Iron: 1.9 mg

7.13 Quinoa Burrito Bowl

Ingredients

- Two cans of adzuki beans, black beans (15 oz. each can)
- White rice or quinoa: 1 cup
- Fresh juice from two limes
- 4 cloves of pressed garlic
- Four green thinly sliced scallions
- One teaspoon of cumin
- A handful of chopped cilantro

Instructions

- Cook the rice or quinoa. Over low flame, in the meanwhile, warm the beans.

- Add in the cumin, garlic, onions, and lime juice. Let it cook for fifteen minutes.

- When quinoa is cooked, add into two serving bowls.

- Add beans on top, and garnish with cilantro.

Nutrition per serving: Calories: 218kcal | Carbohydrates: 25g | Protein:

4 g | Fat: 0.7 g | Sodium: 192mg | Potassium: 198 mg | Fiber: 2.8g | Sugar: 1.7 g | Calcium: 27 mg | Iron: 3 mg

7.14 Raw Pad Thai Recipe

Ingredients

- A half packet of beansprouts
- Three medium zucchini
- Two spring of green onions, thinly sliced
- Shredded red cabbage: 1 cup
- Three carrots (large)
- One cup of cauliflower florets
- Olive Oil
- One bunch of cilantro, roughly chopped

Sauce

- One clove of pressed garlic
- Tahini: ¼ cup
- Tamari: ¼ cup
- One inch of grated ginger root,
- Honey: 1 tsp
- Unsalted butter: ¼ cup
- Lime or lemon juice: 2 tbsp.

Instructions

- Spiralize the carrots and zucchini into noodles.
- In a bowl, add shredded cabbage, beansprouts, coriander, spring onions, and cauliflower mix well.
- Prepare the sauce by mixing all sauce ingredients in a blender; add water if the sauce is very thick.
- Add the sauce into the bowl and coat everything well.
- Top with chopped coriander and lemon juice.

Nutrition per serving: Calories: 256 kcal | Carbohydrates: 21 g | Protein: 6 g | Fat: 2 g | Sodium: 154 mg | Potassium: 281mg | Fiber: 4 g | Sugar: 2.5g | Calcium: 21 mg | Iron: 1.2 mg| phosphorous: 121 mg

7.15 Savory Wrap

Ingredients

- ¼ chopped red onion
- One butter lettuce bunch
- One teaspoon of chopped basil
- One tomato: sliced, chopped
- loosely packed ¾ cup of spinach (leach it)
- One teaspoon of chopped cilantro
- Salt & black pepper

Instructions

- Lay lettuce leaf flat on a surface, add red onion, basil, tomato, cilantro, add spinach too, sprinkle with salt, and black pepper.
- Fold into a roll.
- Serve and enjoy.

Nutrition per serving: Calories: 99kcal | Carbohydrates: 10 g | Protein: 8g | Fat: 0.7 g | Sodium: 132mg | Potassium: 267 mg | Fiber: 6 g | Sugar: 1.2 g | Calcium: 19 mg | Iron: 1.1 mg| phosphorous 211 mg

7.16 Green Beans & Quinoa Salad

Ingredients

- Green beans: 2 cups
- Quinoa: one cup
- Chickpeas: one can drained
- Fresh parsley

Instructions

- Cook quinoa with two cups of water. Boil it and cover it, cook for 12 minutes.
- Cook until all the liquid is absorbed, fluff with a fork, and turn off the heat, set it aside.
- In a bowl, mix all ingredients with black pepper and salt.
- Serve hot with olive oil and lemon slices

Nutrition per serving: Calories: 211 kcal | Carbohydrates: 15.5 g | Protein: 5.7 g | Fat: 2 g | Sodium: 145 mg | Potassium: 213 mg | Fiber: 4 g | Sugar: 2 g | Calcium: 11.9 mg | Iron: 2 mg| phosphorous 198 mg

7.17 Kale & Golden Beet Salad

Ingredients

Salad

- Green onions, four pieces, cut and chopped
- One bunch of kale, cut into thin strips, de-stemmed
- Carrots: 2 medium
- One yellow bell pepper
- Golden beets: 4 medium

Dressing

- Olive oil: 4 tbsp.
- Dried oregano: 2 tsp.
- Apple cider vinegar: 4 tbsp.
- Juice of a half lemon
- One-inch peeled & minced piece of ginger
- Tahini: 3 Tbs.
- Dried basil: 1 tsp.
- Three cloves of minced garlic

Instructions

Salad

- In a bowl, add green onions and chopped kale.
- Chop carrots, bell pepper, the beets and very finely in a food processor.
- Add chopped vegetables into green onion and kale.
- Mix well.

Dressing

- In a bowl, add all dressing ingredients and mix well. Or use an emulsion blender(hand-held) till smooth and creamy.

- Add sauce over the salad.
- Chill before serving and enjoy.

Nutrition per serving: Calories: 217 kcal | Carbohydrates: 9.2 g | Protein: 11g | Fat: 1.2 g | Sodium: 132 mg | Potassium: 134 mg | Fiber: 4.3 g | Sugar: 1.8 g | Calcium: 10.3 mg | Iron: 2.1 mg| phosphorous 178 mg

7.18 Apple & Almond Butter Oats

Ingredients

- Green apple(grated): 1 cup
- Gluten-free oats: 2 cups
- Almond butter(raw): 1/3 cup
- One and a ½ cups of soy milk
- Half tsp of cinnamon

Instructions

- In a bowl, add milk, almond butter, add oats, and mix. Add in the grated apple.
- With plastic wrap, cover the bowl and refrigerate it overnight.
- Add coconut milk if oats become too thick.
- Top with cinnamon powder and serve

Nutrition per serving: Calories: 176 kcal | Carbohydrates: 8.9 g | Protein: 12.4 g | Fat: 1.99 g | Sodium: 121 mg | Potassium: 210 mg | Fiber: 4.3 g | Sugar: 2.7 g | Calcium: 21 mg | Iron: 1.4 mg| phosphorous 92 mg

7.19 Blueberry Pancakes

Ingredients

- Blueberries: 1/3 cup
- 1 and 1/4 cup of homemade almond milk
- Honey: 3 tbsp.
- Grapeseed oil: 2 tbsp.
- One pinch of sea salt
- 1 and 1/2 cup of spelt flour
- For serving, use extra fruit and Agave syrup

Instructions

- In a bowl, mix date sugar and flour, mix well, so no lumps remain. Add grapeseed oil, walnut milk in the flour, and date sugar mixture.
- Whisk it but do not over mix.
- Fold in the blueberries but maintain the lumps. Be careful to not over mix
- Let the griddle preheat to 350 F add a light coating with grapeseed oil.
- Add 1/4 cup of batter on the griddle in the desired shape.
- Cook until bubbles form and edges are brown
- Flip it and let it cook for 1 minute or 2.
- Top with extra fruit and agave syrup, and enjoy.

Nutrition per serving: Calories: 182 kcal | Carbohydrates: 12.4 g | Protein: 6 g | Fat: 2 g | Sodium: 121 mg | Potassium: 112 mg | Fiber: 3.2 g | Sugar: 2.1 g | Calcium: 15 mg | Iron: 1.9 mg| phosphorous 171 mg

7.20 Blueberry Delight Smoothie

Ingredients

- Flax seeds(ground): 1 tbsp.
- Blueberries: half cup
- Hemp seed powder: 1 tbsp.
- Chia seeds: 1 tbsp.
- Soy milk: one cup
- Almond butter(raw): one tbsp.-optional
- Oil: 1 tbsp.

Instructions

- Place all the ingredients in the food blender.
- Pulse on high until well combined and smooth.
- Enjoy

Nutrition per serving: Calories: 89 kcal | Carbohydrates: 7.1 g | Protein: 22 g | Fat: 1.45 g | Sodium: 106 mg | Potassium: 98 mg | Fiber: 3.9 g | Sugar: 1.2 g | Calcium: 11 mg | Iron: 2 mg| phosphorous 87 mg

7.21 Blood Orange, Carrot, & Ginger Smoothie

Ingredients

- One blood orange: peeled and diced
- Almond, coconut or cashew milk: 2 cups
- Pineapple: half cup
- One knob of one inch: minced fresh ginger
- One frozen banana
- One carrot peeled and diced (medium-sized)
- Add in half apple, de-seeded and peeled
- One scoop of vegan collagen: it is optional

Instructions

- In a food blender, add all the ingredients
- Pulse on high for almost one minute, until smooth and creamy.
- Serve with fresh basil leaves on top.
- Enjoy.

Nutrition per serving: Calories: 72 kcal | Carbohydrates: 6.5 g | Protein: 11 g | Fat: 1 g | Sodium: 104 mg | Potassium: 102 mg | Fiber: 5.6 g | Sugar: 1.4 g | Calcium: 21 mg | Iron: 2 mg| phosphorous 112 mg

7.22 Cleansing Detox Soup

Ingredients

- Vegetable broth or water: 1/4 cup
- Turmeric: 1 teaspoon

- Half of red onion, chopped
- Three stalks of chopped celery
- Three chopped medium carrots
- Two cloves of pressed garlic
- One head of small broccoli, cut into florets
- Chopped tomatoes: 1 cup
- Ginger: 1 tablespoon, peeled and freshly minced
- Cayenne pepper: 1/8 teaspoon, or to taste
- Cinnamon: 1/4 teaspoon
- Purple cabbage: 1 cup, diced
- Freshly ground black pepper, sea salt, to taste
- Water: 6 cups
- Kale: 2 cups, stem removed and torn into pieces
- Juice from half of a small lemon

Instructions

- In a big pot, over medium flame, add the vegetable broth. Once the broth is warmed, add in the garlic and onion. Cook for two minutes. Add the fresh ginger, broccoli, carrots, tomatoes, and celery.
- Cook for another three minutes. Add more water or broth if required. Add in the cayenne pepper, turmeric, cinnamon—season with pepper and salt.
- Lower the heat and let it simmer for 15 minutes. Cook until vegetables are tender.
- Add in the cabbage and kale.
- In the end, add lemon juice, let it simmer for 2-3 minutes.
- Turn off the heat
- Serve hot with fresh basil leaves.

Nutrition Per Serving: Calories 139|Fat 1g|Saturated Fat 1g|Sodium 41mg|Potassium 219mg|Carbohydrates 8g|Fiber 2g|Sugar 2g|Protein 3g|Calcium 77mg| iron 1mg|phosphorus 111 mg

7.23 Arugula & Strawberry Salad with Cayenne Lemon Vinaigrette

Ingredients

Salad

- Arugula: 2 cups,
- Walnuts (Toasted)-optional
- Diced apples: 2 tablespoons
- Three strawberries cut into slices
- Blueberries: 1/4 cup

Dressing

- Agave syrup: 1/4 teaspoon or another sweetener
- Extra virgin olive oil: 2 tablespoons
- Powder cayenne pepper: 1/8 teaspoon

- Pinch of salt
- Lemon juice: 2 teaspoon
- Freshly ground black pepper

Instructions

- In a bowl, add all the dressing ingredients, whisk to combine, and set it aside.
- In another big bowl, add all the salad ingredients, pour the dressing all over, and top with toasted walnuts.
- Serve right away and enjoy.

Nutrition Per Serving: Calories 127|Fat 0.9 g| Sodium 137 mg| Potassium 121 mg|Carbohydrates 7g|Fiber 2g|Sugar 1.4 g|Protein 4 g|Calcium 87 mg| iron 1mg|phosphorus 102 mg

7.24 Asian Cucumber Salad

Ingredients

- Grated ginger: 1 tbs.
- Key lime juice: 3 tbs.
- Half tsp. of date sugar
- Powdered, granulated seaweed: 1 tbs.
- Sea salt: 1/4 tsp
- Olive oil: 1 tbs.
- Sesame seeds: half tsp.

Instructions

- In a big bowl, add all the ingredients. Mix them well.
- Serve with your favorite dressing.

Nutrition Per Serving: Calories 121|Fat 0.8 g |Sodium 37 mg|Potassium 108 mg|Carbohydrates 5 fiber 2.3g|Sugar 1.8 g|Protein 4 g|Calcium 88 mg| iron 1.2 mg|phosphorus 89 mg

7.25 Triple Berry Smoothie

Ingredients

- One burro banana
- Strawberries: half cup
- Agave syrup, to taste
- Blueberries: half cup
- Water: one cup
- Raspberries: half cup

Instructions

- Add all ingredients in a food blender.
- Pulse it on high until smooth and creamy. Serve and enjoy.

Nutrition Per Serving: Calories 121|Fat 0.7 g| Sodium 31 mg| Potassium 102 mg|Carbohydrates 7.8g|Fiber 3 g|Sugar 1.2 g|Protein 4.4 g|Calcium 89 mg| iron 1.3 mg|phosphorus 92 mg

7.26 Mushroom Risotto

Ingredients

- Rice: 2 cups
- Olive oil: one teaspoon
- Four mushrooms
- Half onion
- Cayenne pepper, to taste
- Homemade vegetable broth: 4 cups

- Sea salt, to taste

Instructions

- In a large pot, sauté mushrooms and onions in grapeseed oil over medium heat. Cook for 5 to 7 minutes or until mushrooms are lightly browned, and liquid is evaporated, stirring occasionally.

- Stir in rice and cook an additional minute.

- Add in the vegetable broth and additional sea salt and pepper. Cover and cook on a low-heat setting for about 2 hours and 45 minutes or on a high-heat set about 1 hour 15 minutes or until rice is tender.

- Serve hot and enjoy.

Nutrition Per Serving: Calories 312|Fat 1.4 g| Sodium 89 mg| Potassium

128 mg|Carbohydrates 23 g|Fiber 2.9 g|Sugar 2 g|Protein 10 g|Calcium 87 mg| iron 1.3 mg|phosphorus 109 mg

7.27 Green Falafels

Ingredients

- Half cup of flour

- Beans, dry garbanzo (chickpeas): 2 cups

- Red bell pepper: 1/3 cup, diced

- Oregano: 1/4 teaspoon

- Fresh basil: 2/3 cup

- One large onion, diced

- Olive oil for frying

- Half cup of fresh dill

- Sea salt: one teaspoon

Instructions

- Boil the chickpeas, drain the water and wash them.

- In a food processor, add the chickpeas with the rest of the ingredients: flour, sea salt, onion, fresh herbs, red bell pepper, and oregano.

- Pulse on high until all things are finely diced and like coarse. Toss with the spoon and pulse again, taste it, and adjust the seasoning if required.

- Move this coarse meal mixture to a big mixing bowl, use your clean hands, shape them into balls or discs like structure. Place all the balls over parchment paper.

- Put in the refrigerator for one hour to chill.

- You can rather fry these falafels in one inch of oil in a deep pan. Or air fry them at 380 for ten minutes, until golden brown.

- Serve them with your favorite dipping sauce.

Nutrition Per Serving: Calories 276|Fat 1.4 g| Sodium 76 mg| Potassium

145 mg| Carbohydrates 20.3 g| Fiber 2.9 g| Sugar 1.7 g| Protein 8.9 g| Calcium 89 mg| iron 1 mg| phosphorus 87 mg

7.28 Creamy Kamut Pasta

Ingredients

Pasta

- Box of Kamut Spirals: 1 and a half cups
- Dried tarragon: 1 tablespoon
- water:6-8 cups, (to boil your pasta)
- Olive oil: 2 tablespoon
- Onion powder: 1 teaspoon (no salt)
- Sea salt: one teaspoon

Creamy Sauce

- Half medium onion: diced
- Olive oil: divided, two tablespoon
- Sea salt + plus a half teaspoon
- Water: 2 cups
- Freshly ground black pepper
- Sliced baby Bella mushrooms: 2 cups
- Chickpea flour: 1/4 cup
- Almond milk: one and a half cups
- Dried tarragon: 1 tablespoon
- Tomatoes(Roma), chopped 2-3
- Dried oregano: 1 teaspoon

- Onion powder: 2 teaspoon
- Fresh kale: 2 cups packed
- Dried basil: 1 teaspoon

Instructions

Pasta

- In a pot, add water with salt over high heat. Let it boil
- When the water has boiled, add pasta. Cook until tender to your preference.
- To enhance flavor, add seasoning while the pasta is still warm, add onion powder, sea salt, dried tarragon, and grapeseed oil.
- Taste the pasta and adjust the seasoning.

Creamy Sauce

- In a pan, add one tbsp. of grapeseed oil, over medium flame, heat for one minute
- In the hot oil, add in the sliced mushrooms and chopped onions. Stir often let it cook, until vegetables are tender for about five minutes.
- Add in the fresh ground black pepper and salt, 1/4 teaspoon of each. Add in chickpea flour and another one tbsp. of olive oil.
- Mix constantly flour with the oil and vegetables for at least one minute. Flour should not be left dry as it will help thicken the sauce.

- Then add in the can coconut milk, dried oregano, onion powder, half a teaspoon of sea salt, dried tarragon, spring water, half a teaspoon of black pepper dried basil. Mix it well. Let it simmer, uncovered for 20 minutes. Or until sauce becomes thick.

- Then add in the kale, tomatoes, and seasoned, cooked pasta. Cook until the kale is wilted for five minutes. Turn off the heat.

- With time, the sauce will become thicker from the pasta.

- Serve with fresh basil leaves and enjoy.

Nutrition Per Serving: Calories 326|Fat 3 g| Sodium 98.2 mg| Potassium 119 mg| Carbohydrates 25 g| Fiber 2.4 g| Sugar 1.5 g| Protein 22 g| Calcium 43 mg| iron 2.1 mg| phosphorus 102 mg

7.29 Vegetarian Kebabs

Ingredients

- Olive oil 1 tbsp.

- 1 dried parsley, teaspoon

- 2 spoonsful of water

- Two sweet peppers

- Two peeled red onions

- Two zucchinis shaved

Instructions

- Chop the onions and sweet peppers into medium-sized squares.

- Cut the zucchini.

- String the skewers with all the vegetables.

- Then combine the olive oil, dried parsley, wine, and balsamic vinegar in a shallow dish.

- Spray with the olive oil mixture on the vegetable skewers and switch to the hot oven 390F grill.

- Fry the kebabs on each side for three minutes just until the vegetables are light brown.

Nutrition Per serving: 88 calories|2.4g protein|13g carbohydrates|3.9g fat| 3.1g fiber| Potassium 102mg |phosphorous 87 mg

7.30 Carrot Cakes

Ingredients

- One cup of grated carrot

- Semolina 1 tablespoon

- Two egg whites

- One teaspoon of seasonings Italian

- Olive oil 1 tablespoon

Instructions

- Comb the grated carrot, semolina, egg, and Italian seasoning in a bowl and mix.

- Warm the pan with sesame oil.

- With the help of Two spoons, make the carrot cakes and place them in the skillet.

- Fry the patties on each side for four minutes.

Nutrition per serving: 70 calories|1.9g protein| 4.8g carbohydrates|4.9g fat| 0.8g fiber| Potassium 89mg|phosphorous 78 mg

7.31 Vegetables Cakes

Ingredients

- Two cups of mushroom, sliced
- Three cloves of sliced garlic
- One tbsp. of dill dry
- One beaten egg or egg alternative,
- 1/4 cup of cooked rice
- olive oil 1 tablespoon
- 1 chili powder teaspoon

Instructions

- In the mixing bowl, add the mushrooms.
- Add the chili powder, garlic, dill, egg, and rice.
- Mix for ten seconds
- Heat the sesame oil for 1 minute after that.
- Shape mushroom cakes of medium size and put them in the hot olive oil.
- Cook the mushroom cakes on a medium flame for 5 minutes per side.

Nutrition Per serving: 103 calories|3.7g protein|12g carbohydrates|4.8gfat| 0.9g fiber| 41mg calcium| Potassium 92 mg |phosphorous 76 mg

7.32 Glazed Eggplant Rings

Ingredients

- Three sliced eggplants
- One tbsp. of honey
- One minced ginger tsp
- Lemon juice 2 teaspoons
- Three tbsp. of olive oil
- 1/2 teaspoon cilantro
- Water 3 tablespoons

Instructions

- Use ground coriander to rub on the eggplants.
- And heat the olive oil for 1 minute in a pan.
- Add the diced eggplant and organize it into one layer when the oil is hot.
- Fry the vegetables on one side for 1 minute.
- Place the eggplant in a dish.
- Then fill the pan with honey, ginger, lemon juice, and water.
- Get it to a simmer and add the eggplants that have been prepared.
- Cover the vegetables well with the sweet liquid and cook for two more mints.

Nutrition per serving: 136 calories|4.3g protein|29.6g carbohydrates|2.2g fat| 15.1g fiber| Potassium 87mg |phosphorous 81 mg | sodium 109 mg

7.33 Sweet Potato Balls

Ingredients

- One cup of mashed, baked sweet potato, leached
- One tbsp. of chopped fresh cilantro
- One egg alternative
- Three tablespoons oatmeal
- One teaspoon paprika ground
- 1/2 teaspoon of turmeric
- Two spoonsful of olive oil

Instructions

- Mix the egg, ground oatmeal, paprika, sweet potato, fresh cilantro, and turmeric in the cup.
- To make the tiny balls, whisk the mixture once soft.
- Warm the saucepan with olive oil.
- Add the sweet potato balls whenever the oil is hot.
- Cook them until their golden brown.

Nutrition per serving: 133 calories|2.8g protein| 13.1g carbohydrates|8.2gfat|2.2g fiber| calcium 41mg| Potassium 86 mg|phosphorous 78 mg |sodium 103 mg

7.34 Chickpea Curry

Ingredients

- One 1/2 cup of boiled chickpeas
- One teaspoon of powdered curry
- 1/2 teaspoons of garam masala
- Kale, 1 cup
- One tsp of olive oil
- 1/4 cup of soy milk
- 1 tbsp. of tomato paste (no salt)
- Half of a cup of water

Instructions

- Warm the saucepan with oil.
- Add garam masala, curry powder, soy milk, and tomato paste.
- Stir till the batter is smooth, then take it to a boil.
- Add water, chickpeas, and kale.
- Mix and shut the lid on the meal.
- Cook it over medium flame for five minutes.

Nutrition per serving: 145 calories|8 g protein| 15.1g carbohydrates|4 gfat|3 g fiber| calcium 35 mg| Potassium 96 mg|phosphorous 81 mg |sodium 101 mg

7.35 Quinoa Bowl

Ingredients

- 1 cup of quinoa
- Two Cups of Water
- Red bell peppers: 1 cup, chopped
- 1/2 cup cooked rice
- One tbsp. of juice from a lemon

- 1/2 lemon zest teaspoon, grated
- Olive oil 1 tablespoon

Instructions

- Mix the water and quinoa, then cook for fifteen min. Then detach it from the heat and allow for ten minutes to rest.
- Move your cooked quinoa to a large bowl.
- Add the sweet pepper, sugar, lemon juice, olive oil, and lemon zest.
- Stir the mixture well in the serving bowls.

Nutrition per serving: 290 calories| 8.4g protein| 49.9g carbohydrates| 6.4gfat| 4.3g fiber| trans-fat 0mg| Potassium 88mg |phosphorous 71mg|sodium 100 mg

7.36 Vegan Meatloaf

Ingredients

- One cup cooked chickpeas
- 1 onion, diced
- 1 tbsp. flax seeds ground
- 1/2 teaspoon chili flakes
- 1 tbsp. olive oil
- 1/2 of a cup of carrot, diced
- 1/2 cup stalk of celery, chopped
- 1 tbsp. of tomato paste, no salt added

Instructions

- Warm the saucepan with olive oil.
- add the carrot, celery stalk, and onion. Cook for ten minutes or until the vegetables are tender.
- Chickpeas, ground chili flakes, flax seeds are then added.
- With the electric mixer, mix the combination until creamy.
- Later, with baking paper, cover the loaf mold and move the blended paste inside.
- Add tomato paste and scatter.
- Bake the meatloaf for twenty minutes in the oven and bake at 365 F.

Nutrition per serving: 162 calories|7.1g protein| 23.9g carbohydrates 4.7g fat|7g fiber|transfat 0mg| Potassium 88mg|phosphorous 69 mg|sodium 103 mg

7.37 Vegan Shepherd Pie

Ingredients

- 1/2 cup cooked quinoa
- 1/2 cup puree red bell pepper
- 1/2 of a cup of carrot, diced
- 1 minced shallot
- 1 tbsp. olive oil
- 1/2 cup of potato, baked, mashed
- 1 chili powder tsp
- 1/2 cup sliced mushrooms

Instructions

- In a frying pan, place the carrots, shallots, and mushrooms.

- Apply coconut oil and fry the veggies once tender but not fluffy, for ten minutes until its tender.

- Then combine the cooked vegetables with the tomato puree and chili powder.

- Move the paste and flatten even into the casserole shape.

- Cover the vegetables with mashed potatoes afterward. Contain the shepherd's pie with a baking sheet and bake 25 minutes in the preheated 375 F oven.

Nutrition per serving: 136 calories|8.2g protein| 20.1g carbohydrates|4.9gfat| 2.9g fiber| Potassium 93.2 mg |phosphorous 87mg|sodium 104 mg

7.38 Vegan Steaks

Ingredients

- 1-pound head of cauliflower

- 1 tsp turmeric

- 1⁄2 cayenne pepper teaspoon

- Olive oil: 2 tablespoons

- 1⁄2 teaspoon powdered garlic

Instructions

- Rub with cayenne pepper, ground turmeric, and garlic powder and slice the cauliflower head into the steaks.

- After which line the cookie sheet with baking paper and put the Cauliflower steaks in place.

- Spray with olive oil and cook for 25 minutes at 375F just until the veggie steaks are gentle.

Nutrition per serving: 92 calories| 2.4g protein| 6.8g carbohydrates| 7.2g fat|3.1g fiber| Potassium 85 mg |phosphorous 78 mg|sodium 93 mg

7.39 Quinoa Burger

Ingredients

- 1/3 cup cooked chickpeas

- 1⁄2 cup cooked quinoa

- 1 tsp of Italian seasonings

- Olive oil: 1 tsp

- 1⁄2 of an onion, diced

Instructions

- In a food processor, pulse the chickpeas on high, until smooth

- Then combine the quinoa, the Italian seasonings, and the grated onion with them. Till densely concentrated.

- Shape the burgers from the combination after this and position them in a lined baking tray.

- Spray olive oil on the quinoa burgers and cook them for twenty minutes at 275 F.

Nutrition per serving: 158 calories|6.4g protein| 15.2g carbohydrates|3.8g fat| 4.7g fiber| Potassium 78 mg |phosphorous 67 mg|sodium 92.3 mg

7.40 Stuffed Sweet Potatoes

Ingredients

- One sweet potato (leached)
- ¼ cup whole-grain penne pasta
- 1 tsp tomato paste
- Olive oil 1 tsp
- ¼ teaspoon minced garlic
- 1 tbsp. soy milk

Instructions

- Break the sweet potato in two and stab it 3-4 times with a fork.
- Spray the sweet potato halves with olive oil and cook in the Preheated to 375 F oven for about half an hour or when the vegetables are tender.
- In the meantime, mix up penne pasta, tomato paste, minced garlic, and soy milk.
- Whenever the sweet potatoes are baked, spoon out the vegetable meat and spice it up with a penne pasta combination.
- Cover the sweet potatoes with the pasta mix.

Nutrition per serving: 105 calories| 2.7g protein| 17.8g carbohydrates| 2.8g fat|3g fiber| Potassium 87 mg| phosphorous 66 mg |sodium 85 mg

7.41 Tofu Masala

Ingredients

- Tofu 1 cup, minced
- 1/2 cup of almond or soy milk
- 1 tsp of garam masala
- Olive oil for 1 tsp
- 1 tsp paprika ground
- 1/2 cup of red bell peppers, sliced
- 1/2 onions, sliced

Instructions

- In a frying pan, heat the olive oil.
- Add chopped onion and fry till light brown.
- Put the ground paprika, tomatoes, and garam masala in the mixture. Get it to a boil
- Add soy milk and whisk thoroughly. Let it boil for five minutes.
- And add sliced tofu and cook for three minutes with the food.
- For ten minutes, leave the cooked meal to rest.

Nutrition per serving: 155 calories|12.2g protein|20.7g carbohydrates|8.4g fat| 2.9g fiber| Potassium 78 mg|phosphorous 71 mg|sodium 94 mg

7.42 Tofu Parmigiana

Ingredients

- One cup of firm tofu, cut finely

- One olive oil tsp
- 1 tsp tomatoes sauce (no salt)
- 1/2 teaspoon Italian seasonings

Instructions

- Combine the tomato sauce and Italian seasonings in a mixing dish.
- Then add the cut tofu well with the tomato mix and leave to marinate for ten minutes.
- Heat the olive oil, too.
- Place the sliced tofu in the hot oil and roast it on each side for three minutes or until the tofu is golden brown.

Nutrition per serving: 83 calories|7g protein|1.7g carbohydrates| 6.2g fat|0.8 fiber| calcium 34 mg| Potassium 67 mg |phosphorous 56 mg|sodium 76 mg

7.43 Vegan Stroganoff

Ingredients

- Two cups of sliced mushrooms
- 1 tsp of wheat whole-grain flour
- 1 tsp olive oil
- 1 minced onion
- 1 dry tsp of thyme
- 1 clove of garlic, diced
- 1 black pepper ground tsp
- 1/2 cup of almond milk

Instructions

- Warm the saucepan with olive oil.
- add the onion and mushrooms and cook them for ten minutes. Stir the vegetables. From time to time,
- Spray them with ground black pepper, thyme, and garlic after that.
- Take the mixture to a boil and incorporate soy milk.
- Add the flour, now whisk thoroughly until it is combined.
- Heat the stroganoff mushroom until it becomes thick.

Nutrition per serving: 70 calories|2.6g protein| 6.9g carbohydrates| 4.1 fat|1.5g fiber| calcium 34 mg| Potassium 78mg |phosphorous 65 mg| sodium 87 mg

7.44 Vegan Croquettes

Ingredients

- One peeled, boiled eggplant
- Two potatoes, mashed (leached)
- Almond meal: 2 tablespoons
- 1 tsp pepper chili
- Olive oil: 1 tsp
- 1/4 teaspoon nutmeg

Instructions

- Mix the eggplant, with the mashed potato, coconut oil, chili pepper, and ground nutmeg.

- From the eggplant combination, make the croquettes.
- Warm the skillet with olive oil.
- Place the croquettes in the hot oil, then fry them on each side for two minutes until its light brown.

Nutrition per serving: 180 calories|3.6g protein| 24.3g carbohydrates| 8.8g fat|7.1g fiber| calcium 54mg| Potassium 87 mg|phosphorous 81 mg|sodium 93 mg

7.45 Stuffed Portobello

Ingredients

- Four Mushroom caps Portobello
- 1⁄2 zucchini, grated
- 1 onion, sliced
- Olive oil
- 1 tsp
- 1⁄2 teaspoon of dry parsley
- 1⁄4 teaspoon of garlic, minced

Instructions

- Combine the diced tomatoes, rubbed zucchini, dry parsley, and ground garlic in a food processor.
- And fill the mushroom caps with the blend of zucchini and move them to the baking paper tray.
- Cook the vegetables till they are cooked through or for twenty minutes.

Nutrition per serving: 84 calories|14 g protein| 10.3 g carbohydrates| 1.3 g fat| 0.9g fiber| Potassium 65 mg |phosphorous 66 mg |sodium 78 mg

7.46 Chickpeas Stir Fry

Ingredients

- One cup of garbanzo, cooked
- One zucchini, diced
- One cup of mushroom cremini, chopped
- One tablespoon olive oil
- One tsp: black pepper ground
- One tablespoon fresh, minced parsley
- 1 tsp of juice from a lemon

Instructions

- Warm the saucepan with olive oil.
- Stir in the mushrooms and cook for ten minutes.
- And add the cooked garbanzo beans and zucchini. Whisk the ingredients well enough and cook them for an extra ten minutes.
- Sprinkle the vegetables with ground black pepper and lemon juice. After this, for five minutes, cook the meal.
- Add and blend the parsley. Heat it for an extra five minutes.

Nutrition per serving: 231 calories|11.3g protein|33.9g carbohydrates| 6.6g fat| 9.6g fiber| potassium 78 mg

CPSIA information can be obtained
at www.ICGtesting.com
Printed in the USA
LVHW020906270521
688665LV00014B/650